PANS, CANS, ...& AUTOMOBILES

A Comprehensive Reference Guide for Helping Students with PANDAS and PANS*

*Pediatric Autoimmune Neuropsychiatric Disorders Associated with Streptococcal Infections and Pediatric Acute-onset Neuropsychiatric Syndrome

Jamie F. Candelaria Greene, PhD, BCET

First Edition Design Publishing
Sarasota, Florida USA

PANS, CANS, ...& AUTOMOBILES

ISBN 978-1506-902-21-0 – HC/CL
ISBN 978-1506-901-87-9 PRINT
ISBN 978-1506-901-86-2 EBOOK

LCCN 2016936853

June 2016

Published and Distributed by
First Edition Design Publishing, Inc.
P.O. Box 20217, Sarasota, FL 34276-3217
www.firsteditiondesignpublishing.com

Author Photograph by Alanna M. Greene

These materials are intended to provide academic and informational resources only. Opinions expressed are those of the author unless otherwise cited. Moreover, information included in this book should not be considered as a substitute for medical, legal, psychiatric, or psychological advice from a qualified provider. Regarding the specific needs of any one individual, it is advised that readers contact their respective resources to address any educational, legal, medical, psychological, and psychiatric aspects that are of concern.

Library of Congress Cataloging-in-Publication Data Candelaria Greene, Jamie Fitch

PANS, CANS, ...& Automobiles / written by Jamie Fitch Candelaria Greene.
p. cm.
ISBN 978-1506-901-87-9 pbk, 978-1506-901-86-2 digital

1. MEDICAL / Pediatrics.

P196

To Alanna

The Perceiver

Acknowledgements

I am so grateful to the many who made this book possible. To Diana Pohlman (Executive Director Emeritus of Pandasnetwork.org) for her encouragement to assemble this work; to Amy Fishman Smith, RN, NP and Dr. Sunjya Schweig, who offered hope, healing, and wonderful insight regarding the manifestations of this illness; to Ann Honigman DC, MPH, who traveled this journey with me from the beginning; to Dorothy Duff Brown PhD, my friend and editor, who stayed by my side during the initial drafts of the work; to Frank C. Worrall PhD (UC Berkeley) who was good enough to facilitate my Visiting Scholar Researcher position (2013-2015); to Mary F. Candelaria PsyD and Linda C. Avery PhD, for offering such critical support and feedback on PANS psychiatric aspects, and to Sr. Madeleine Hanot (Daughters of the Cross of Liege) for her vision and example.

To my parents, Jo C. and James Fitch, whose empathy towards others was so pivotal in the makings of my world perspective; to my mother, who by example, urged me to show up and not 'shut-up;' to my father, the best teacher of special education I will ever know, whose compassion and belief in the rights of all students to be educated resulted in one of the first public special education programs in the US; and to my brothers and sisters, for their limitless support, compassion, brilliance, and love.

I am deeply thankful to the many who took the time to offer valuable information and feedback on various sections of the work, specifically, Drew Maxwell, Amaryllis Case RN, Anne Beireis (Student Advocate), Mary Ellen Quinn RN, Barbara A. Dimopoulos MA (LD Specialist), Alison Angell RN, Jodi Biskup RN, Stephanie Holeva MA, Diana Pohlman, Amy Fishman Smith RN, NP, Ann Honigman DC, MPH, Jerome F. Candelaria, Linda Morales MA, Cheryl Theis MA (DREDF), Helena Fitch-Snyder MS (UC Davis), Tiffani Maxwell, Mark Anderson OD, Pia Lingstrom OD and Mark Wu OD (UC Berkeley School of Optometry), staff from The California State Department of Education (Special Education), David Grisham OD, Joe Feldman (CASE), Celine Forte RN, and those equally helpful others who wished to remain anonymous. Also, for their superb help with the book's graphics design, I would like to thank Reese Bretow, Colin Yeo, Liem Nguyen, Lillian Almohajer, Jackie Guo, and Andrea Szeto.

To the wonderful parents and providers who were willing to share their experiences with me during my term as a Visiting Researcher Scholar, I am so indebted to you; and, of course, to the brave survivors of this illness who offered their insights- you truly light the way forward for the rest of us.

And to others who added their actions and voices of wisdom and insight along the way: Dan and Pat Fitch, Wade Frazier, Lori Candelaria, Will Snyder, Nino Hernandez, Jon Ishibashi, Marty Beane, Neal Adams, Mel Lum, Martin Fong, Cynthia Kunisaki, Dr. Larrie Goldsmith, Joy Dean, Michael Lee, Dr. Glynda Hull, Dr. Anne Haas Dyson, Dr. Denise Herd, Dr. Robert Costa, Laura Leahy, Michael Hans, Griff Hodge, John Carbon, Lance Smith, Brad Thomas, Ann Esparza, Peter and Kathryn Hill, Stephen Ramos, Janice Quan, Melanie S. Weiss RN, Parissa Khosh, Judith Duhl, Robert Ithurburn, Diane Alexander, Christopher Honeywell, Paul Gross, Pat Schmitz, Carrie Blanche, Evan Lee, Dr. Sean McPhetridge, Miriam Lenhardt, Alvin Ludwig, Kimberly Kennedy, Madelyn Merola, Carmel Zimmerman, Faye Wong Chow, Rebecca Shoshan, Sarah Johnson, Eliseo Baca, Nirmala Mallipatna, Joe Pearse, Dr. William Durbrow, Beverly Marks, Vatiri de Karisoke, Ngugi Harrison, Barbara Conlon, Marian B. Candelaria, Joan Ralph, Eric Shawn, Antoineta D'Costa, Heather McCracken Wu, Captain Philip Smith, Dr. Patricia Rice Doran, Sr. Patricia Ainsworth, Dr. Lester Isenstadt, Dr. Leo Cheng, Dr. Janice Tona, Sr. Elena Pettenuzzo, Dr. Susan Swedo, Dr. Miroslav Kovacevic, Dr. Dritan Agalliu, Dr. Beth Latimer, Dr. James Leckman, Dr. Wayne Goodman, Dr. Eric Storch, Dr. Tanya Murphy, Brenda Ramirez-Paulino, Vickie Blavat, Vicki Savitt, Millie J. Moran, Dr. Kate C. Larson, Jenny Sui, Dr. Diana Pandell, Lauren Balk, Donna Konuch, Paige Rich, Emily Klein, Maria Nagy, Dr. Brad Berman, Dr. Michael Torres, Elizabeth Dandenell, the gracious Carlos Santana, the Barr family, the Davis family, the Tsutsui family, the Wu family, the Neff family, Raquel Diaz, Jessica Simpson, the Rodriguez-Hall family, and the Tezdogan family.

Lastly, I am grateful to my husband, Jay "Al" Greene, for his generous spirit, and for his belief in me and in this work.

To my precious children- you have been by far my greatest and best adventure. Thank you for your encouragement, and for your gifts of love and time.

...Finally, to my beloved son - Hand in hand, you took me on a path I did not think I wished to take; and yet, the journey would ultimately bestow strength, wisdom, and kindness in its wake, and that is all grist for the good.

TABLE OF CONTENTS

PREVIEW

From the fall of 2013 to the fall of 2015, I had the fortunate opportunity of being a Visiting Researcher Scholar at the University of California at Berkeley. My aim was to gather as much information as I could regarding the educational implications of the multifaceted condition I knew to be PANS (Pediatric Acute-onset Neuropsychiatric Syndrome). Toward these efforts, I interviewed parents, providers, educators, administrators, educational advocates, programs specialists, PANS survivors, and others. This work is the result of what was gleaned during those interviews and research, where resulting information would, in the end, validate prior notions of pedagogy, and reshape others.

The intent of this book is to provide information to those who are the primary 'stake-holders' in the educational care and support of students with PANS. For this reason, the material is geared toward those in the educational field, but also to providers who seek information about the educational ramifications of PANS on their patients, and, of course, to families and loved ones who are seeking similar help for their child.

A few words about the organization of this book may be helpful. The sections, as well as the reference section and appendices, are developed to be relatively independent resources that one can refer to when needed. Citations and notes can be found at the end of each section. Bolded words will usually signify key terminology, such as that used in Education, Psychology, and Medicine. Finally, at the onset, I must freely confess to the probable overuse of italicized words, which are done in an attempt to signify concepts of special significance.

Section I provides a general overview of PANDAS, PITANDS, PANS, and the lesser known, CANS. Inherent in the discussion of these medical diagnoses is nothing short of a whirlwind medical history lesson, where parent demand, as well as devoted and caring providers and researchers, propelled desperately needed research into PANS and its treatment. Section I details the mechanism by which PANS occurs, the areas of the brain that are affected, and the types of function that these areas of the brain are associated with.

Section II takes us to the *Learning Environment.* This is usually in the classroom. However, it can also be on the playground, at the beach or the state capital (if on a class field trip), or even at a *Homecoming* game, - anywhere that a student's same-aged curriculum is expected to occur. Whereas Section I introduces the reader to what we know about PANS' impact on behavior, attention, and learning skills, Section II describes what a careful observer might notice, in terms of how it can manifest in various 'classroom' settings. It also addresses the critical roles that *Executive Functioning* and *Language* play in the educational experience of students with PANS.

How might the school 'culture' and staff dynamics of a particular school and school district impact the recognition, formal identification, and delivery of educational services for students with PANS, and how can loved ones and providers effectively begin to move forward towards the appropriate educational program and treatment? More importantly, what is the academic 'big picture' here? Section III allows us to take a reflective pause before jumping directly into a plan of action. This section details how PANS is strikingly different from other disabling conditions that school districts tend to be familiar with. It lays the preplanning/groundwork down, which will be vital later on when considering what educational avenues would, and would not, serve to support these students' unique educational needs.

There is the realm of *Medicine*. There is the realm of *Psychology*. And there is the realm of *Education*. Each has their own culture, language, hierarchy, and related laws. As families and providers shift from the universe of physicians to that of psychiatrists and psychologists, and then to educators, a whole new framework that now includes the delivery of special services and education, comes in to view. Section IV provides us with an example of how *one* country's (US) legislative backdrop serves as a framework, in which *all of its students* can be supported, and their educational opportunities safeguarded. In understanding and recognizing the legal parameters of their country's educational mandate, individuals can begin to take realistic steps to ensure that their student is receiving the most appropriate education, at least within the agreed upon and expected codes of that nation's educational system.

Section V familiarizes the reader with the general processes of obtaining services, accommodations, and modifications to the student's educational day. What should parents reasonably expect to have happen at an educational planning meeting? Who are the 'cast of characters' expected to attend, and why is each important? As one begins to understand the *How's, Who's, Where's*, and *When's* of these educational processes, one can gain a better grasp at not only knowing what to expect during the meetings, but what to expect as *appropriate* in terms of delivery of services (or, when the actual help begins).

In Section VI, we finally come to review actual, specific recommendations for accommodations, testing considerations, compensatory strategies, and supportive services that can help our students succeed as much as possible during treatment, and as they heal. Of course, many students with PANS will share commonalities of educational needs related to the illness. However, each student will have unique needs, too, that will need to be addressed. For this reason, Section VI is designed to offer a *continuum* of suggested services and accommodations, rather than a boiler plate dictum where one-size-fits-all.

Section VII reviews some common themes that emerge as parents, schools, and local jurisdictions strive to serve students with special needs. What may be considered positive indications that the school *is* fostering and safeguarding the type of educational experience that will be *most appropriate* and *least restrictive* for this unique learner? This section includes aspects to consider when gauging the extent to which the needs of all students, but particularly those with PANS, are being addressed and met. It also suggests ways in which community and government agencies can play a greater role in addressing PANS.

Finally, resources and appendices are attached. Resources include a glossary of common terms and acronyms related to the field of Special Education and related services, a reference section, and a list of resources. Appendices include the *Yale-NIMH PANS Scale*, symptoms of OCD and tics, taken from the *Yale-Brown Obsessive-Compulsive Scale (CY-BOCS)* and the *Yale Global Tic Severity Scale (YGTSS)*, respectively. Then, samples of the types of letters (that may be helpful when requesting assistance and services) are included, followed by examples of educational *goals* and *objectives*.

Lastly, it should be acknowledged that, while every effort has been made to address the special learning needs of young people with PANS, the *unique needs of each student* will require that families, schools, and supporting providers look to *their own community expertise*, applicable laws, and guidelines when deciding on educational treatment plans. Moreover, this book merely reflects a 'snapshot' in time. Laws may change, and certainly, our knowledge of PANS will evolve. In this spirit, it is hoped that this work will serve as a springboard, to spark new discussion and treatment options for this clearly, paradigm-changing group of learners.

"*You've got to see it to believe it,*
...and you've got to believe it to see it."

-Amy Joy Fishman Smith

Section I

FROM PETER PAN TO PANDAS AND PANS

By all accounts, Sir JM Barrie, the author of the celebrated children's tale, *Peter Pan*, loved children. A generous supporter of London's *Great Ormond Street Hospital for Sick Children* throughout the late 1800's, he would ultimately bequeath to them the entirety of his Peter Pan royalties. Yet, even in this beloved author's fantastical imagination, he would have no way of foreseeing how his efforts to care for sick children of his day would wend their way into providing critical insight towards the identification of a futuristic syndrome--that would one day come to be called *PANS*.

Mr. Barrie, a compassionate and keen observer of the young, was not unlike an older, even more renowned writer of young heroes and heroines, Charles Dickens. Both Barrie and Dickens (an earlier supporter of the hospital) were products of Victorian England, and both men were sensitive to the plights of children, especially if they were unlucky enough to be born into lives of poverty. The double ravages of malnutrition and child labor would make these children especially vulnerable to nineteenth century scourges. Even when offered the best pediatric care of the time, such as at the Great Ormond, many would be left permanently weakened by infections, or not survive at all. As Hospital archivist Andrea Tanner noted, of all the patients admitted there due to infectious disease between the years 1852 and 1914, only four of five survived.[1]

Still, it can be said that when the Great Ormond opened its doors in 1852, it was the beginning of nothing short of revolutionary care and treatment for desperately ill children. Moreover, it would represent a phenomenal sea change in both the knowledge and effectiveness of pediatric medicine itself. The surge in information- gleaned from the hard work and careful observations of its hospital physicians, nurses, and staff- would change the fates of untold numbers of children, including those youth of the future who would have surely perished without such efforts.

Of course, such potentially deadly illnesses as diphtheria, bronchitis, tuberculosis, and even measles were nothing new to nineteenth century physicians. What *was* new, was the opportunity for this hospital (one of the first pediatric hospitals in the world, and the first in England) to identify clinical syndromes that specifically affected *children*. This was made possible through the availability of "typical clinical cases," whereby large numbers of pediatric patients with similar manifestations of an illness could now be followed. In particular, such complex multi-systemic diseases as **Rheumatic Fever (RF)** could be tracked and categorized.[2 3]

Technically referred to as **Acute Rheumatic Fever (ARF)**, Rheumatic Fever results from an untreated/or uncured Strep infection. Specifically, the triggering agent is a **group A beta hemolytic streptococcal** or **(GABHS)** infection, and it includes **Strep Throat, Impetigo,**[4] and **Scarlet Fever**.[5] Rheumatic Fever is described as a *latent* condition that occurs months after the most obvious symptoms of the GABHS infection.[6] Symptoms can include a rash, fever, and swelling, redness, and pain of the joints (arthritis). Unfortunately, the consequences of Rheumatic Fever can be very serious. One consequence includes the debilitating condition of **Rheumatic Heart Disease (RHD)**,[7] whereby the infection travels to the heart muscle, and the heart valves become inflamed.[8] The resulting **Carditis**[9] that is associated with RHD is known to cause such symptoms as a rapid heart rate, fatigue, and shortness of breath. Moreover, if subsequent infections are left untreated, such accumulative damage to the heart can result in death.

One of the more obvious consequences of Rheumatic fever, however, is **Sydenham's chorea (SC)**.[10] This is a condition that results in involuntary movements that are often described as jerking, rapid, and uncoordinated, and that typically last several months. Sydenham's is associated with other symptoms as well. These include behavior changes (including those associated with **Obsessive Compulsive Disorder (OCD)**, changes in speech (*Dysarthria*), difficulties swallowing (*Dysphagia*)[11], loss of motor skills (including a deterioration in handwriting), headaches, slowed cognition (which includes the ability to think and to process new information), facial grimacing, fidgetiness, and hypotonia (muscle weakness).[12 13]

Most educators, especially in the world's more developed countries of today, would be hard-pressed to *define* Sydenham's chorea, much less recall a student who had it. However, in the last half of the nineteenth century (as in less affluent areas of the world even today), "chorea" was not uncommon to see at all. At the Great Ormond between 1860 and 1900, *chorea* (which comes from the Greek word for 'to dance') was the fourth most frequent cause of illness, and in the 1880's, it temporarily became the second.[14 15]

Careful clinical notes (such those excerpted below) describe one of the milder cases of Sydenham's chorea. These were noted by Dr. Charles West, who was also the founder of the hospital.

Date: *April 4th, 1865* Name: *Alice Pope* Age: *8 years, 4 months*

> *...This is the first attack of chorea. It began in Christmas week. The right arm was first affected. The right leg followed.*
>
> *...Not a very bad case. She can sit up unsupported (and) lay hold of an object with extra hand. She can stand (and) walk unsupported. The right limbs are already more choreal than the left. Tongue protruded easily (and) stayed out without difficulty. ...Mucus membs. rather pale.* [16]

It is true that physicians had been aware of "St. Vitus Dance" since 1686, when Thomas Sydenham, after whom the condition was named, first described it. However, with the study and categorizations of numerous entries, such as the one above, Sydenham's chorea would now become a well-defined nosological (disease) entity.[17] [18] Still, it would not be until the dawn of the twentieth century, that researchers such as F. J. Poynton (also a staff physician at the Great Ormond) would identify the ***streptococcus*** bacteria as the trigger of Rheumatic Fever,[19] thus lighting the way to a more comprehensive understanding of the origin, and links, between infection and behavior.

PITANDS and PANDAS

Let us now fast-forward our story to the latter half of the twentieth century. Thanks to the pioneering work of researchers like those at the Great Ormond, Rheumatic Fever could now be more easily identified, and its infectious agent tested for in the lab. Even better, with the discovery of the usefulness of penicillin in the 1950's,[20] the infection itself could be treated with such medications as antibiotics, and children could be healed.

In previous centuries, parents could only look to their children's outward (and obvious) symptoms to realize that they were ill. For some families, the uncontrolled jerking movements of their child's extremities might have been the only clue that their child had Sydenham's chorea. However, now, pediatric medicine offered much better diagnostic tools to explore, rule out, identify, and if necessary, treat conditions that were not so obvious to the naked eye. Children with suspected Rheumatic Fever, for example, could be examined for Rheumatic Heart Disease too. If diagnosed with it, **prophylactic medications** (such as a continued course of antibiotics) could prevent a subsequent infection from causing further damage to their heart valves.[21]

But by the 1980's, something new was happening in the realm of intense and unexpected behavioral responses to pediatric infection. The National Institute of Health (NIH) in the U.S. became aware of a group of children who began to experience a sudden onset of psychiatric symptoms following infections from a variety of different agents. These included *Streptococcus pygenes,* and also *Varicella* (Chickenpox) and *Mycoplasma pneumoniae* ("Walking pneumonia"). Pioneering researchers first termed this condition **Pediatric Infection Triggered Autoimmune Neuropsychiatric Disorders (PITANDS).** Under this new PITANDS umbrella, the **Group A Streptococcus (GAS)** infections would emerge as the most researched entity, particularly because of its similarities with Sydenham's.[22]

Like Sydenham's, the NIH recognized that with this new condition, such unexpected *symptoms were the result of a pediatric infection* (Strep) that triggered an **autoimmune response**. (This is a term for any response of the host's, or body's, immune system to attack, or turn on, its own tissues, cells, or molecules.)[23] At the same time, however, there were significant *differences* noted between the two as well. First, Sydenham's produced *more motor dysfunction* than this new phenomena did, which generally produced *tics and/or a psychological component* (such as OCD). Secondly, the **latency period** between the infection and the onset of behaviors happened much later in Sydenham's *(6 to 9 months)* in contrast to that of this new group *(days to weeks).*[24]

This particular subgroup of PITANDS became defined by an "acute prepubertal onset of tics or OCD symptoms, association with GAS infection, and specific neuropsychiatric symptoms." [25] [26] [27] It came to be called **PANDAS**, which is the acronym for **Pediatric Autoimmune Neuropsychiatric Disorder Associated with Streptococcus Infections.**[28]

PANDAS is an autoimmune condition, whereby in response to a GAS infection, the body's *own immune system* mistakenly attacks itself along with the GAS, thereby triggering brain/ neurological inflammation, and a host of psychiatric and physical changes that follow. In determining whether or not an individual carried a diagnosis of PANDAS, the following diagnostic criteria were identified:

1. The presence of clinically significant obsessions, compulsions and/or tics often with multiple tics.
2. An unusually abrupt onset of symptoms or a relapsing-remitting course of symptom severity.
3. A prepubertal onset.
4. An association with other neuropsychiatric symptoms.
5. An association with streptococcal infection.[29]

Let us now take a closer look at various aspects of these five diagnostic criteria.

***Number 1**: The presence of clinically significant obsessions, compulsions and/or tics often with multiple tics.*

In this case, the term "**clinically significant**" means that the obsessions, compulsions, and/or tics can be quantified, or measured, and that the resulting rating is significantly above what would normally be expected for that person's peer group (often based on age and gender). Two assessments that are used as measures for these criteria (with examples of symptoms provided in the appendices) are the *Yale Brown Obsessive-Compulsive Scale OCD* (**CY-BOCS**), and the *Yale Global Tic Severity Scale-* (**YGTSS**) to quantify Chronic Tic Disorder.[30]

In the PANDAS/PANS population, there are a wide range of expressions of **OCD** and **Tics**. **Obsessive thoughts** include unwanted and recurrent thoughts, doubts, or images that intrude into one's mind despite attempts to resist or control them.[31] A few examples of **obsessive behaviors** include the fear of contamination and of harming oneself or others.[32] Examples of **compulsive behaviors** include excessive washing, checking, repeating, counting, and ordering. **Tics** can be expressed as **phonic (or vocal) tics**, **motor tics**, or **both**. **Phonic tics** can include such utterances as coughing, throat clearing, barking, or sniffing. Examples of **motor tics** include such unexpected movements as shoulder shrugging, kicking, or facial grimacing. Tics are also described as **simple** (involving just one muscle group) or **complex** (involving multiple muscle groups). **Complex vocal tics**, for example, may involve *more meaningful speech* (such as words or phrases) than **simple vocal tics**. **Complex motor tics** might include facial grimacing, combined with a head twist and a shoulder shrug. In some cases, complex motor tics might even look like the person is doing the tic on purpose.[33]

***Number 2**: An unusually abrupt onset of symptoms or a relapsing-remitting course of symptom severity, and*

***Number 5**: An association with streptococcal infection (as indicated by positive titers on blood or other lab tests).*

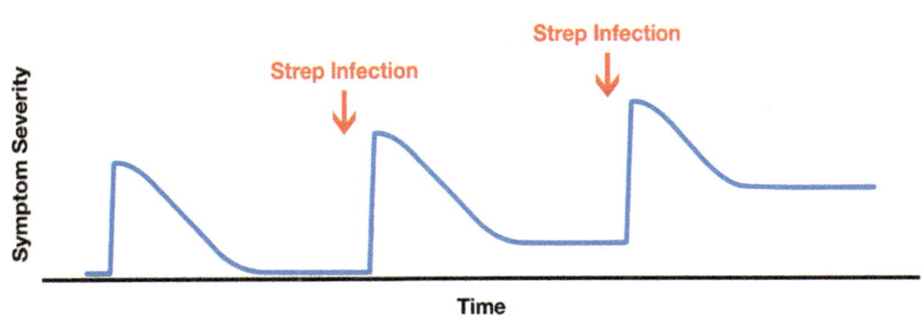

Taken from NIMH Developmental Neuroscience Branch [34]

In the graph above, one can see a visual representation of how symptoms dramatically increase following exposure to the streptococcus infection. (The vertical blue line represents *how severe the symptoms are*, and the flat horizontal line represents *the length of time that the person was monitored*. Notice how after the *first* exposure, the symptom count returns to **baseline**. (Baseline infers that either *no symptoms* have been noted and/or suggest that the individual has returned to whatever was considered pre-PANDAS behavior). However, notice how after each *successive* exposure to infection[35] [36] the symptom count *increases*. Moreover, while it certainly lessens in severity after each illness or exposure, it returns less and less *completely* back to the baseline. (This is one reason why providers consider it be so important to address and treat this illness early on in the disease process.)

Another important consideration is that even **asymptomatic** acquisition of GAS infections can initiate a rise of ASO titers.[37] This suggests that families and schools may not always see outward symptoms of the infection itself prior to the onset of PANDAS behaviors.

Number 3: *Prepubertal onset*

This was included in the criteria, because the typical age of onset is generally recognized to be between four and seven years old.[38] Moreover, it was recognized that there are a number of changes that happen in the immune system at the time of puberty (and into the teen years) that make individuals less likely to develop PANDAS as they get older.[39] [40]

Number 4*: An association with other neuropsychiatric symptoms.*

In addition to tics and obsessive and compulsive behaviors, other significant neurospsychiatric symptoms have also been reported to happen during these PANDAS exacerbations. These include severe **separation anxiety** [41] [42] [43] where, for example, the child might be very "clingy," and have difficulty separating from his/her caregivers or sleeping alone in his room. It could include other symptoms such as **anxiety**, **irritability**, (sometimes with aggression), **emotional lability** (having to do with the control and expression of their emotions), or **depression.**[44] Moreover, indicators of **behavioral/developmental regression** have been noted too,[45] [46] whereby the individual is functioning (socially, motorically, perceptually, emotionally, etc.) like someone much younger. Symptoms of developmental regression can include temper tantrums, and poorer motor skills (such as messier handwriting). However, it can also include a weaker ability to plan and organize their lives, to care for themselves, and to participate in 'social language' with same aged peers. Additional symptoms include hyperactivity, inattention, and fidgetiness.

Moreover, in its review of PANDAS, The National Institute of Health (US) cited more commonly reported symptoms, and these included the following:

- Sleep disturbances, including night terrors and difficulty falling asleep and staying asleep.[47]
- Motoric hyperactivity, abnormal movements, and a sense of restlessness.
- Sensory abnormalities (surrounding light, sound, tactile, olfactory, and kinesthetic awareness).[48]
- Concentration difficulties and loss of academic abilities, particularly in math and visual-spatial areas.[49] [50]
- Increased urinary frequency and a new onset of bed-wetting (including an increased need to use the bathroom during school hours).
- Night- time bed wetting and/or day- time urinary frequency.
- Fine/gross motor changes (e.g. changes in handwriting).
- Joint pains, stiffness, and general lethargy.

(NIMH, 2012) [51]

Lastly, in their seminal study of fifty children with PANDAS, Dr. Susan Swedo and her colleagues reported a number of comormid (or co-occurring) **psychiatric diagnoses** in the patients' histories. These included: Attention Deficit Disorder (40%); Oppositional Defiant Disorder (40%); Conduct Disorder (40%); Major Depression (36%);

Dysthymia (12%); Separation Anxiety (20%); Avoidant Disorder (8%), Overanxious Disorder (28%), Specific Phobia (16%), Eating Disorder (2%), Enuresis (12%), and Encopresis[52] (10%).[53]

Mechanism of the PANDAS Illness

Having looked at the aspects of these diagnostic criteria more closely, what is the ***mechanism*** *and its related elements* that are viewed as the catalyst for PANDAS to occur?

Researchers put forth the following three tenets:

- 1. A **genetic pre-disposition** to an abnormal immune response.
- 2. The **creation of an anti-neuronal antibody**[54] that interferes with normal neuronal *(brain)* activity.
- 3. **A breach in the blood brain barrier**, thought to be due to inflammation, that negatively activates a protein in the brain called **calcium–calmodulin dependent protein Kinase II (CaM Kinase II**), which then allows the entrance of anti-neuronal antibodies. New research states that this breach allows the anti-neuronal antibody to reach neuronal tissue and interfere with neuronal functioning, including increased activation of CaM Kinase II (which is a precursor to dopamine).[55 56]

Regarding this last tenet specifically, researchers such as Dr. Christine Kirvan of California State University, Sacramento,[57] recognized that there was an association between *autoimmune response to GAS infections* (such as Strep), and *brain cells producing too much **CaM Kinase II***. In turn, the release of too much CaM kinase was found to influence changes in levels of **dopamine** in the brain.[58]

Dopamine is one of a number of **neurotransmitters**, or brain chemicals, that communicate information throughout the brain and body. (Neurotransmitters are responsible for relaying signals between **neurons** (nerve cells), and they help to facilitate a number of bodily functions, including appetite, sleep, hormone release, and energy levels. They also play an important role in regulating mood and thought processes, and are involved in our ability to focus and remember things.) Dopamine, in particular, is associated with motor control and feelings of pleasure and reward. It is also a prominent neurotransmitter involved in the efficient functioning of the brain's **basal ganglia**,[59 60] (which will be discussed further along in this section). Two commonly known medical conditions associated with both the basal ganglia and inefficient levels of dopamine are **Huntington's disease**[61 62] (characterized by uncoordinated and jerking movements/chorea and changes in cognition), and **Parkinson's disease** [63 64] (associated with muscle rigidity, tremors, and a slowing down of physical movement).

When researchers examined and compared levels of CaM Kinase II and **neuronal antigens** (or **anti**body **gen**erators) in children with PANDAS and Sydenham's Chorea, they found *higher* levels of CaM Kinase II, along with elevated titers, or measures, of antibodies[65] against lysoganglioside,[66] Tubulin,[67] dopamine D2 receptor,[68 69 70] and dopamine D1 receptor.[71] Researchers also confirmed, through blood tests, that CaM Kinase II activation levels in PANDAS patients were, in fact, ***lower*** than what was seen in those with Sydenham's chorea. At the same time, however, these levels were ***much higher*** than what was observed in children with *non*-PANDAS related ADHD, Tourette Syndrome, or OCD.[72]

The *Cunningham Panel* was named after Dr. Madelyn Cunningham of the University of Oklahoma, who spearheaded the effort to develop a commercially available test to measure CaM Kinase II and the neuronal antigens noted earlier in suspected PANDAS patients. For many families struggling with a child suffering from PANDAS, results from the Cunningham Panel would become another important data point in providing validation regarding the presence of brain inflammation in their children.[73]

Tonsils, Mice, Our Sense of Smell, and PANDAS

Important research continues to unlock the mysteries of the PANDAS mechanism. Recently, groundbreaking research has brought us even closer to our understanding of how autoantibodies can cross the otherwise *leak-proof* **blood-brain barrier** (**BBB**), and result in the type of immune response and inflammation seen in PANDAS.[74] [75] [76] Researchers, led by Dr. Dritan Agalliu of Columbia University Medical Center (CUMC), and Dr. Patrick Cleary at the University of Minnesota, reported that Streptococcal A-specific immune cells, called ***Th17*** **cells**, were found in the tonsils of individuals exposed to GAS (Group A Strep) infections (including individuals with PANDAS). Their team then studied the tissues of mice that were infected intra-nasally with Strep A. This resulted in the finding that Th17 immune cells were able to reach the brain by traveling along the surface of **olfactory** (odor-sensing) axons.[77] These particular axons extend from the nasal cavity through the **cribriform plate**, which is a thin, sieve-like, (porous) bone that separates the nasal cavity from the brain. These scientists showed that from there, the Th17 cells were able to reach the **olfactory bulb** in the brain, where sensory information about odors is processed. As Dr. Agalliu explained in a related CUMC Newsroom online article,[78] *"Once these Th17 cells enter the brain, they break down the blood-brain barrier, allowing autoantibodies and other Th17 cells to enter the brain and promote neuroinflammation."*

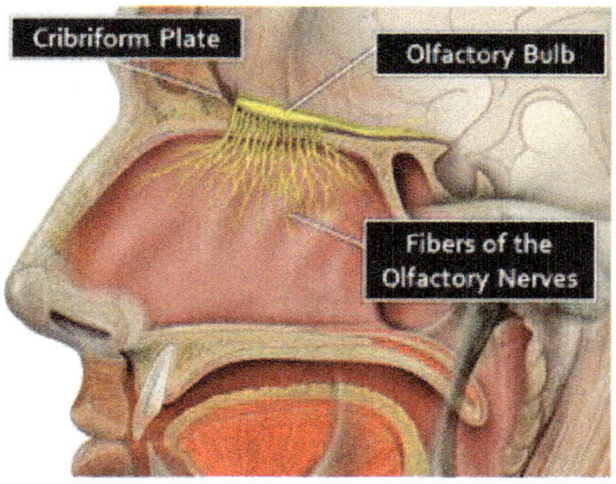

As these findings shed light on how infection plays a role in the mechanism of PANDAS, they also hold promise for developing new ways to diagnose, monitor, and treat this illness too. Moreover, such research extends similar hope in allowing for a better understanding of *other autoimmune diseases* that affect the central nervous system too, such as rheumatoid arthritis and multiple sclerosis.

From PANDAS to PANS

Spurred on by the dedicated efforts of parents and organizations, such as *pandasnetwork.org*, research and practice evolved and progressed more rapidly with every passing year. Providers and researchers began to notice, for example, that individuals with the outward symptoms of PANDAS did not always have a history of GABHS infections, or necessarily other illnesses associated with PITANDS. In 2011, **CANS** (Childhood Acute Neuropsychiatric Symptoms),[79] and ultimately, ***PANS*** *(***Pediatric Acute-onset Neuropsychiatric Syndrome**[80] were terminology that were used to describe the similarity in mechanism, without (necessarily) an apparent GABHS involvement.

PANS substantially expanded the umbrella of possible triggers leading to the kind of abrupt and dramatic behaviors seen in PANDAS. Within the broadened scope of PANS, **Infectious Triggers** such as GAS infections (PANDAS) were acknowledged as possible triggers to the onset of such symptoms, but other microbes too, such as Lyme and Mycloplasma (that include "Walking pneumonia") were acknowledged as well. Moreover, PANS now included **non-infectious triggers** as well, such as environmental factors, metabolic disorders, and other factors, including immunodeficiency, etc. Specifically, PANDAS is now considered to be a subset of PANS.[81]

Table I: Hierarchy of the Pediatric Acute onset Neuropsychiatric Syndrome

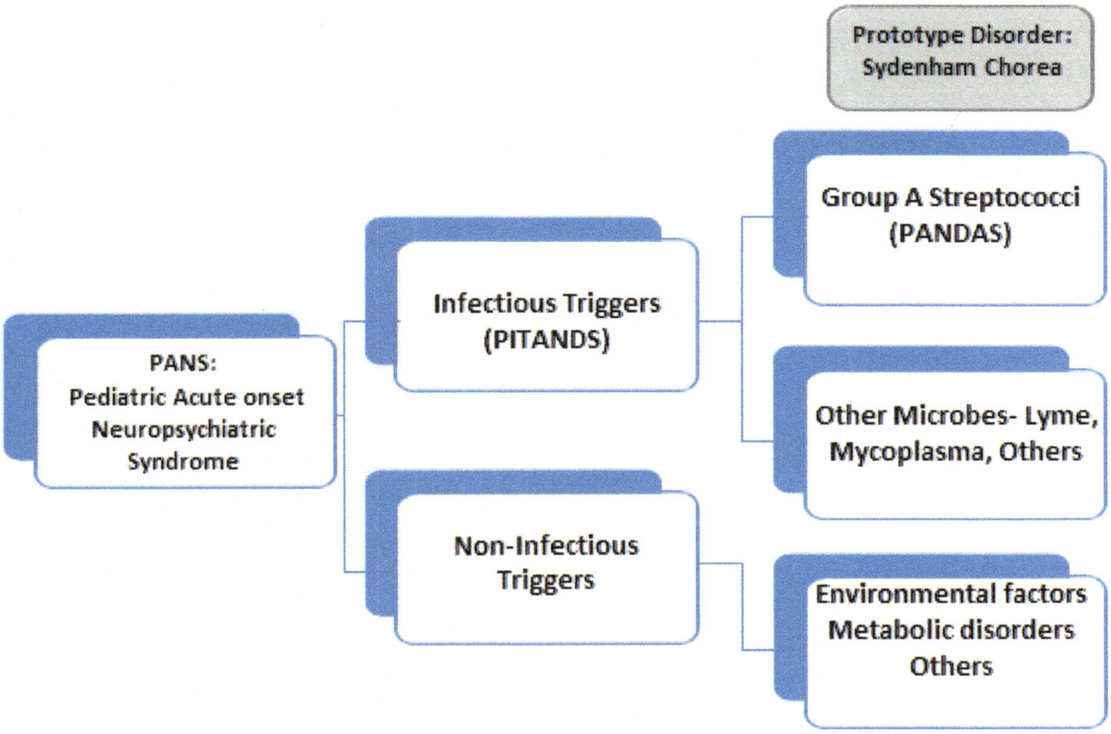

Table taken from: Swedo SE, Leckman JF, Rose NR (2012) From Research Subgroup to Clinical Syndrome: Modifying the PANDAS Criteria to Describe PANS (Pediatric Acute-onset Neuropsychiatric Syndrome). Pediatrics and Therapeutics 2:113. doi:10.4172/2161-0665.1000113

Experts who convened at the National Institute of Health in 2010 produced a list of **diagnostic criteria for PANS**, and this was defined as follows: (Notice how the key descriptors of PANS- of which PANDAS is a subset- are *acute* and *multifaceted*.

I. Abrupt, dramatic onset of obsessive-compulsive disorder or severely restricted food intake.
II. Concurrent presence of additional neuropsychiatric symptoms (with similarly severe and acute onset) from at least two of the following seven categories
   1. Anxiety.
   2. Emotional lability and/or depression.
   3. Irritability, aggression and/or severely oppositional behaviors.
   4. Behavioral (developmental) regression.
   5. Deterioration in school performance (related to attention-deficit/hyperactivity disorder [ADHD]-like symptoms, memory deficits, and cognitive changes).
   6. Sensory or motor abnormalities.
   7. Somatic signs and symptoms, including sleep disturbances, enuresis or urinary frequency.
   8. Symptoms are not better explained by a known neurologic or medical disorder, such as Sydenham's chorea.[82 83]

Along with these diagnostic criteria, these experts pointed out that PANS is a *"diagnosis of exclusion."* This means that other known medical diseases have to be ruled out first, before a diagnosis of PANS can be given. Secondly, they acknowledged that a number of PANS symptoms will, by definition, *overlap with such psychiatric disorders* as OCD, depression, and Tourette Syndrome, etc.). In determining then whether the patient has PANS, the litmus test is: Can the symptoms be described as "**acute-onset in multiple domains?**"[84] In other words, do the symptoms come on suddenly, and do they affect the individual in a number of areas of function, (such as noticeably poorer hand writing, unexpected physical movements, *and* OCD symptoms)?

Diagnosis, Treatment, and Prevalence

Diagnosis: Of course, along with meeting the diagnostic criteria presented earlier, a diagnosis of PANS warrants a very comprehensive diagnostic evaluation. In 2015, in a consensus statement of experts that was presented in the *Journal of Child and Adolescent Psychopharmacology*, the following components of a systematic evaluation were recommended. These include a family history, patient medical history and physical examination, psychiatric evaluation, mental status examination, general laboratory studies, infectious disease evaluation, evaluation for autoimmune and auto-inflammatory diseases, testing for neural autoimmunity, evaluations for immunodeficiency, and additional diagnostic evaluations (such as brain MRI's, sleep studies, etc).[85]

Treatment: The team of researchers who contributed to the consensus article on PANS [86] pointed to the future as ultimately leading to "empirically based algorithms for (both) diagnosis and treatment." In the meantime, however, once a diagnosis of PANDAS/PANS is made, treatment generally focuses on correcting the condition that was responsible for triggering the inflammation response.[87] [88] It is generally acknowledged that the earlier treatment is sought, the more rapidly the child has a chance for a full and complete recovery. In the case of infections, this may include antibiotics or antiviral medications. Moreover, prophylaxis with antibiotics may be used to decrease streptococcal infections and neuropsychiatric symptom exacerbations among children in the PANDAS subgroup. [89] In more severe cases, plasma is used to provide **Intravenous immunoglobulin G** (**IVIG**) [90] [91] and **Plasmapheresis** (PEX).[92] [93] Other medications that might be used include steroids and non-steroidal anti-inflammatory Drugs (NSAIDS).[94]

Whereas neuropsychiatric medication may also be attempted to treat corresponding symptoms, the general rule of thumb is to *"start low and go slow,"*[95] in that as a group, this population is observed to be very sensitive to such psychotropic medications[96] (as indicated by a preponderance of corresponding negative side effects that have been reported). Strategies provided through behavioral therapies, such as cognitive behavioral therapies (CBT) have been shown to be effective in some children, and helpful to families struggling with facets of the illness.[97] [98]

At the same time, (for long term sufferers of this condition, especially) treatment from other specialties have been sought to alleviate or address related symptoms. Along with primary intervention coming from physicians, nurse practitioners and other providers (who specifically address the PANS itself) families have sought help from others. These include physical, occupational, educational, and speech therapists, along with practitioners in the fields of Psychology, Psychiatry, and Chiropractic, Homeopathic, Naturopathic, and Acupuncture medicine.[99]

Prevalence: Through their arduous collection of feedback from 700 families, *pandasnetwork.org* [100] was able to glean the following information about a large group of affected children. First of all, they found that the **age of onset** for the children who were ages 1 to 3 years was *11%, for* ages 10 to 13 years- *19%*, and for children 14 and over, a very low *1%*. The largest age group (69% of affected children) experienced their first onset of symptoms between 4 to 9 years old. Moreover, on their website *(pandasnetwork.org)*, they included Dr. Susan Swedo's research findings of the first fifty children, that confirmed a younger age of onset- 6.5 (plus or minus 2 years) if the youngster's primary symptom was tics, and 7.4 (plus or minus 2 years) if it was OCD. They also reported Dr. Swedo's findings regarding a higher ratio of boys to girls, especially below the age of 8.[101]

In terms of actual numbers of PANS sufferers, the true prevalence of PANS is difficult to ascertain, as it is likely underreported. However, *pandasnetwork.org* estimates the number to be at least 1 in every 200 children.[102] This estimate builds upon the research of Dr. Swedo, who attributes PANS to approximately 25 percent of children diagnosed with OCD and tic disorders, such as Tourette's syndrome. [103]

PANS Related Symptomatology and Its *True* Prevalence in the Schools

It is important to take a momentary pause to consider the actual prevalence of youth in our schools who may, in fact, be struggling with PANS. This is important, because whether the illness is *medically diagnosed or not*, it is the *school* (and, of course, the family), that face the deleterious consequences of PANS on a day-to-day basis. Put another way, outside of the immediate family, *the public school system will be the primary entity that ends up 'holding the bag'* when it comes to addressing manifestations of this illness, at least during the school day.

Let us return to the estimate of 1 in 200 hundred children- What does this mean, in terms of *actual numbers of* students, for the schools that serve them?

To put this into perspective, let us first highlight figures submitted for other, more well-known disabling conditions of school-aged youth:

- <u>Diabetes</u> under aged 20: About 208,000, or *1 in 400* in this age group.[104]
- <u>Legal blindness</u> among students aged 21 and younger: 60,393.[105]
- <u>Childhood cancers</u> (including all cancers): About 15,780 were expected to be diagnosed with cancer in 2014, and *1 in 285* were expected to be diagnosed with cancer sometime before the age 20.[106]

Clearly then, even a conservative incidence of 1 in 200 youth would far surpass in numbers those being served from such "low-incidence"[107] disabling conditions as those listed above, and others, such as cerebral palsy and deaf-blindness.

US public schools, like others in most 'developed' areas of the world, are charged to address students' symptoms and behaviors as they affect their academic needs and participation. This is true *whether or not* their families can afford (or access) the appropriate medical care and testing needed to diagnose and treat PANS. In the meantime, (and certainly at PANS' worst), families, teachers, and others will have daily, if not hourly proof, evidenced by the child's behavior alone, that something is terribly wrong. Given the urgent need to act in response to such symptoms, most will take immediate steps to take corrective, or at least, *accommodative* actions. Moreover, in many cases, such short-term measures may be offered or treated under (technically) *other* medical, psychiatric, or educational 'umbrellas.'

This means that for many students affected by PANS, *the lack of a formal PANS diagnosis will not necessarily mean that their debilitating symptoms are not being noticed or accommodated for.* In conversations with seven parents and four young adult 'survivors' of this illness, for example, a "lag time" existed of between one and nine years, between initial symptoms of PANS and diagnosis.[108] During this time, students were accommodated for, both *informally*, and *formally* (through written educational agreements). Such measures took place in the classroom, in resource rooms, in home/hospital tutoring, and in **Bridge** programs (designed to strengthen social and organizational skills). Prior to any official diagnosis of PANDAS/PANS then, these services were provided under the rubric of *other conditions* that provided eligibility. These included conditions such as ADHD, anxiety, Tourette Syndrome, or other psychiatric or medical diagnosis.[109]

However, these students were some of the 'lucky' ones, in that they had *two things* going on in their favor; two critical safeguards- that would provide, at the very least, *adequate* educational interventions that would keep the student 'afloat.'

<u>*First, They Had at Least One Parent Who:*</u>

1. Had the *interest, time, opportunity, and resources* to address the child's needs.
2. Was *knowledgeable* that the behaviors and learning impairments were (or possibly were) medically or psychologically based.
3. ***Either*** *held the diagnostic "proof,"* (through doctors letters, etc.) that confirmed at least one medical or psychological diagnosis (that would provide eligibility for services, and guide the school in setting appropriate accommodations and assistance)-

   Or, *provided communications* to the effect that these *diagnoses were being explored/ruled out.*

4. Had the *language skills* to effectively communicate this (and the corresponding need for interventions and services) to the educational staff.

Secondly, They Had the Support of Key Members on Their Child's School Staff Community (Including Both Instructors and Administrators) Who:

1. *Accepted and acted on parental feedback and concerns* (in terms of establishing a rationale for interventions and other services).
2. *Supported the implementation of modifications and services* for the student, based on:
   - An established diagnosis, *or*
   - An interim plan for services (while additional testing was being conducted).
3. *Thought 'outside the box.'* If additional testing did not reveal a definitive diagnosis, or confirm other criteria needed for eligibility for school services, these staff would consider *other avenues to secure help* for the student. (In other words, the *diagnosis* did not drive the call for educational services, *the student's limitations and needs did.*[110]

The advantages noted above are instructive to point out, in that they often play critical roles in how appropriate academic assistance for any one student is obtained, but especially one with a novel type of illness such as PANS. However, a compelling question emerges regarding the fates of other students, who may not have these advantages. What happens, if, for example, a student shows up to school with debilitating PANS symptoms, and his family has *no knowledge* of its medical origin, nor *access* to the appropriate medical care to diagnose or treat it? What happens if he is not one of the *'lucky'* ones, who has both a parent and school staff member who will knowledgably and effectively advocate on his behalf? Certainly this student's behaviors, absences, and failures will be addressed in some way, but how? Just as importantly, how will the *lack of* a *diagnosis of PANDAS or PANS* affect the conversation surrounding the student's behavior, motivation, character, abilities, and intelligences?

Two Recurrent Themes in the Study of PANS: The Basal Ganglia and Molecular Mimicry

PANS and the Basal Ganglia

The anatomic area of the brain that is most implicated in PANS is said to be the basal ganglia.[111] [112] *Ganglia* are masses of nerve cells. Located deep in the upper third area of the brain referred to as the **forebrain** area, the basal ganglia's relay function allows for strong, efficient interconnectedness among different areas of the brain. These areas include the **cerebral cortex,** which is associated with thought and action, and includes creativity, planning, language, and perception.[113] Other parts include the **thalamus** (involved in the relay of most sensory and motor information, as well as in the regulation of sleep states, consciousness, and alertness),[114] and the **brainstem** (involved with numerous integrative functions, including heart rate, breathing, sleeping, and eating).[115] Other significant areas include the **hypothalamus,** which constantly receives input from different parts of the brain, and plays an important role in the body's hormonal system and the expression of emotion,[116] and the **olfactory bulb**, which plays an important role in our sense of smell (and, as it turns out, in the mechanism of PANS itself).[117] Lastly, the **frontal lobe** (not to be confused with the forebrain), is the section of the cerebral cortex specifically associated with such feats as reasoning, movement, planning, language, and emotions. It is just one of four sections, or **lobes** of the cerebral cortex that also include the **parietal lobe**, the **occipital lobe**, and the **temporal lobe**.

As noted earlier, the neurotransmitter **dopamine** features prominently in the smooth functioning of the basal ganglia, most notably in an area called the **striatum,** which receives input from the cerebral cortex.[118] [119] Two other areas of the basal ganglia include the **globus pallidus**, which *transmits* messages to the thalamus, and the **substantia nigra** (an area that plays an important role in reward, addiction, and movement). The substantia nigra, in turn, *sends and receives* messages to the **stratium.**[120] [121] [122] [123]

The critical switching station nature of the basal ganglia allows for efficient learning and memory, and facilitates the ability to manage emotions, movement, and sensory information. At the same time, the basal ganglia also plays an important role in routine behaviors or habits[124] and language processing.[125]

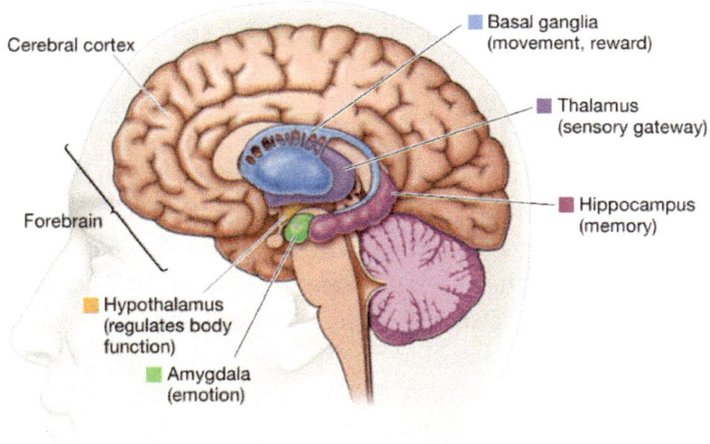

(credit studyblue.com)

Still another important feat of the basal ganglia surrounds one's ability to *inhibit,* or control, *unwanted* muscular activity that would interfere in the execution of a purposeful movement.[126] For example, if a person wanted to write a word with a pencil, he would first relay messages to the appropriate muscles to reach for the pencil, and then to hold/constrict his fingers and hand muscles around that pencil (and at just the perfect amount of tension). Next, the basal ganglia would orchestrate the fluent movement of the fingers and hand to *write the word*. However, as this feat is being carried out, the basal ganglia would also work *to prevent other muscles from making movements* that would interfere with this process. It is thanks to the basal ganglia that for most people, the final writing product looks fluid, neat, and, most importantly, legible.

Of particular relevance to reading and writing skills, too, the basal ganglia play a fundamental role in eye movements.[127 128 129] The fluent decoding and comprehension of text, numbers, and other images normally proceeds so efficiently for most people, that its process is not only rarely questioned, but assumed. In reality, however, the skill of reading is an incredibly complex feat of the human brain.

The processing of text, like the processing of human faces, entails a series of **saccadic** eye movements[130 131] (or micro movements) across the visual field. When reading, for example, the eye will stop briefly, to 'fixate' and perceive a new image of text through the retina, before instantly moving on to the next image of text.[132] (Technically, one perceives and makes meaning of text only after the eye has completely stopped moving.) Fortunately, for most people, such masterful orchestration of the basal ganglia, in conjunction with other parts of the brain, allows for effortless execution of this skill. (Among other areas of the brain, these include the **occipital lobes**, which are responsible for the processing of visual information.) [133 134]

It is no wonder then, that dysfunctions of the basal ganglia can be associated with a number of deficits surrounding reading[135] and number processing.[136] As Dr. Tanya Murphy and her colleagues point out in the consensus statement issue of 2015 regarding the characterization of the PANS phenotype,[137] **visual processing deficits** are a primary area of difficulty in this population.[138 139] Such impairment would predictably threaten a number of other related activities too, such as reading, handwriting, physical activity, visual memory, etc.

<u>PANS, the Basal Ganglia, and Behavioral Dysfunction</u>

Of course, for families who live with the cataclysm of PANS' intense and disruptive behaviors on a daily basis, the 'inflammation of the basal ganglia' represents more than just a regression in academic skills. Its dysfunction can represent the crux of survival itself.

This is because these youth suffer from the disadvantages of having a <u>multi-system *illness*</u> **and** an <u>*immature*</u> ***and*** <u>*jeopardized brain*</u>, specifically in the area associated with attention, planning, decision making, and self-control. Normally, the **prefrontal cortex** of the frontal lobes (closest to the forehead and associated with such **executive**

function) does not even reach maturity until the very late 20's.[140] Moreover, the *younger* the person is, the more he relies on other parts of his brain for decision making, such as the **amygdala.** Part of the **Limbic system**, the amygdala, associated with the processing of emotions and emotional responses, is more fully formed (respectively) than the frontal lobes--all throughout childhood and adolescence.[141] Predictably then, especially as symptoms worsen and the emotion-based *"fight or flight"* amygdala continues to carry significant weight in their decision making, these children's reactions to upsetting triggers may lack the thoughtful self-control that would otherwise help them regulate their responses.[142] Especially if they are already in a state of reactivity, or having a *flare*, they will now have even *less* access to the "executive function" area of their brain (that would provide the critical *'Aim'* segment of the *Ready/Aim/Fire* process of decision making).

Tragically then for this youth and his family, this triple-pronged debilitation involving thwarted basal ganglia can mean this: Not only will the sufferer be wracked with anxiety, OCD, tics, and other debilitations. He will also *lack sufficient cognitive recourse/remedies* (by way of limited access to his critical *'higher thinking'* brain areas) that would otherwise *help* him constructively deal with these fears, misperceptions, worries, and discomfort.

At the same time, this signals something else too, especially for loved ones and providers who are desperately trying to cope with the challenging behaviors associated with this illness. It is that commonly held beliefs, regarding what many view as *"appropriate responses to such behaviors"* (such as time outs, verbal admonishments, and especially physical punishment) serve to only heighten emotional responses in these children. As emotional flares are fueled even further, such reprimands and punishments can predictably become ineffective at best, and detrimental at worst.[143]

PANS and the Phenomena of Molecular Mimicry

Just as it is believed to play a strong role in the mechanism of Rheumatic Heart Disease (where Strep is able to take on the appearance of look-alike proteins in heart tissue) and Rheumatic Fever related joint inflammation (where Strep is similarly able to take on the appearance of joint tissue), **Molecular Mimicry** is assumed to play a similar role in the development of PANS too.

In PANDAS, for example, if a vulnerable individual contracts Strep, it may be possible that the initial infection may contain a *"super antigen"* that is not easily eradicated with antibiotics. (New research also indicates that at times, the Strep may hide in the crypts of the tonsils and adenoids, further exacerbating symptoms[144]). Whatever the exact causation, however, PANDAS autoimmune episodes derive from what Strep specialists call "**the molecular mimicry theory**." During an infectious episode in a susceptible person, the autoimmune system mistakenly attacks the host's brain cells, thereby opening the blood brain barrier, and *"settling in"* to the host tissue of the brain (i.e., the basal ganglia).[145] [146] As a result, the person's own (misdirected) antibodies end up attacking not only the triggering agent (Strep), but also the neighboring (look alike) areas of the brain too.[147] [148] The inflammation process occurs then, *exactly where it is not supposed to-* in the individual's own tissue and organs. When molecular mimicry involves the heart and joints, this inflammation process can lead to heart damage and arthritis, respectively.[149] In PANDAS or PANS, it leads to a specific set of psychiatric, behavioral, and other associated health symptoms.

This mechanism of molecular mimicry figures prominently into why parents and providers of children with PANDAS are so concerned about repeated exposures to Strep or other infectious diseases, and therefore, why they need to know about possible exposures in the class. Even if the child appears asymptomatic, she can still have been exposed to enough of the 'triggering' agent (such as Strep or Mycoplasma) to precipitate a new onslaught of symptoms.

From the Halls of the Great Ormond to the Halls of the NIH: Coming Full Circle in the Research, Diagnosis, and Treatment of a New Multi-systemic Disease Called PANS

Let us now return to those early pediatric hospitals of the nineteenth century, such as the Great Ormond of J M Barrie's *Peter Pan* fame. The new availability of large amounts of clinical notes on the same condition allowed researchers to discover that in pediatric illnesses, as in adult-onset illnesses, there are a number of variations within one disease entity. Within fifty years of The Great Ormond's Street Hospital opening its doors to children, a number of unexpected and welcomed discoveries surfaced. A case in point surrounded one of the top pediatric complaints of its day, 'chorea.' (Sydenham's) chorea would eventually be identified as just *one* presentation of Rheumatic Fever, along with inflammation of the joints and Rheumatic Heart disease, for example. Moreover, over time, these large numbers of case histories would offer the opportunity to confirm *variations within variations* of the illness too (such as mild/ moderate/severe levels of jerking, degree of speech impairment, or degree of psychological manifestation, etc.) Along with the level of impairment, other variables, including formerly unrecognized areas of psychological or physical systems affected, identification of a triggering agent, and effective modes of treatment, would finally be revealed.

Similarly, as the number of youth with PANS continues to grow, information gleaned from these patients and their families will continue to accumulate, and researchers will have more opportunities to recognize the many variations within which PANS is expressed- not withstanding its symptoms, host vulnerabilities, triggering agents, treatment options, etc.[150]

Dr. Tanya Murphy and her colleagues, in the groundbreaking (2015) collection of journal articles that focused on PANS, provide an elegant example of this. Her findings first detail the more commonly seen manifestations of the affected group. She reports for instance, how all of the respondents cite high levels of anxiety and emotional lability, as well as relate comparatively low evaluations regarding their quality of life. She also goes on to report that, of the forty-three youth studied (aged 4-15), most exhibited visual spatial impairment, separation anxiety (77%), generalized anxiety (47%), school avoidance (47%) and clinically significant depressive symptoms (nearly 25%). [151]

However, she then reaches further in her delineation of symptoms, as she presents three distinct symptom clusters that emerged from this study. The first cluster of the three, operationally defined as "**Core Characteristic PANS Symptoms,**" includes emotional lability, anxiety symptoms, sleep disturbances, deterioration in school, and behavioral regression. The second cluster, "**Streptococcal symptoms,**" includes urinary symptoms, ADHD, handwriting deterioration, sensory problems, and simple tics. Finally, a third cluster, "**Cytokine-driven,**" include those symptoms that are often described as part of *cytokine- induced sickness behavior* (having to do with behavioral changes in humans and animals following infection). These include food restriction, mydriasis (pupil dilation), fatigue, gastrointestinal problems, depressive symptoms, elevated Mycoplasma (which includes 'Walking pneumonia'), hallucinations, and /or psychotic symptoms, and complex tics. [152]

Another elegant example illustrates how this expanse of knowledge surrounding PANS etiology, not only confirms what we know about this condition, but reaches out to illuminate our understanding of conditions such as OCD and chronic tics. In their research, Dr. Carol Cox and her colleagues focused on a group of youth, ages 4-27 years, who had suffered chronic tics and OCD for at least a year. They also had a known (or possible) history of streptococcus infection too. These researchers then compared their findings (drawn from blood samples) of this group, to that of groups of youth who were in the following groups: 'healthy controls;' strep-*negative;* youth with OCD only; and youth with tics only.

Their results indicated that indeed, there was strong evidence that among the 222 youth who had a *combination* of strep infection, tics, and OCD especially, there was a significant association of related symptoms along with accompanying anti-neuronal antibodies and increased CaMKII levels. In other words, going beyond those youth already identified with PANDAS/PANS, there is emerging evidence that *immunological and infectious etiology may play a strong role in conditions that have often been thought to be solely 'psychiatric' in nature*, such as OCD and tics. This, in turn, will have profound implications for the way we view, understand, treat, and hopefully, heal such conditions in the future.

In this way, our understanding of the PANS phenomena continues to grow, as studies like those of Dr. Murphy, Dr. Cox, and others, continue to reveal the nature of PANS in greater depth and breadth.

The Important and Evolving Role of the Parent as Team Member in the Medical Treatment of Children

Along with the growing availability of new case histories that allows researchers to examine PANS more fully, something else has come forward in the study of 21st century research on pediatric illnesses. It is the emerging voice of the parent- as an advocate, as a mediator, and as a manager, of course; but just as importantly, to our understanding of how the illness actually manifests -notably outside of the relatively sedate clinical setting-, as an 'authority.' Without this critical input and partnership on the part of parents, substantial gains made in the area of identification and treatment of this multi-systemic, complex disease would surely be stunted.

It can only be assumed, or at least hoped for, that in previous eras, for example, parental input did play a role in the review of a child's medical history, confirmation of symptoms, and access to appropriate treatments, and records. However, it is fair to say that comparatively little was *codified,* in terms of specifically stating what these parental rights and access to services and records *were*. (Historically speaking, as we shall see in Section IV, this is not altogether unrelated to the mirrored stance regarding the parental role in education too.)

There has arguably been, no other time to date when parents have had potentially more *access* to medical services, *collaboration* with providers, and actual *control* (backed up by laws) regarding the medical care of their children. Clearly, with such a debilitating illness as PANS, where the child is *absolutely* unable to obtain treatment and (fully) identify symptoms on his own, the voice of a parent should be as welcomed as it is necessary.[153]

Of course, obstacles to obtaining appropriate medical care still exist for way too many families (as confirmed by the important work of Diana Pohlman[154] of *pandasnetwork.org,* and noted PANDAS author and advocate Beth Maloney[155]). Still however, regarding medical care of their children, many countries of the 21st century *do* at least recognize legally some degree of parental input and rights. For example, parental authority is commonly acknowledged when their written consent is required for impending care, treatment, and participation in medical research. The importance of the parental voice is further reflected in **formal diagnostic tools** too. These include such standardized measures given to assess the levels of their child's behavior, and related measures associated with levels of family stress and burden of the illness, such as the **Caregiver Burden Inventory.**[156] **Informal intakes** of medical history, status of symptoms, and responses to treatment continue to rely on the essential perspective of the parent as well.

Such empowerment and acknowledgement of the parent as 'team member' benefits everyone; - most importantly the child, of course, but also the family, and within a much larger scope, what we know of this formidable condition itself. For as an active participant in the management of her child's health needs, the parent brings to the table an expertise of a subject matter that no one else will ever know in such depth- her child. This knowledge of the *whole child*, (both seen and unseen by others) serves to ultimately give back to science a deepened, layered understanding of this truly astonishing phenomena.

Let us now step away from the clinical setting, to where most students spend the prime of their day- the learning environment; usually in a classroom, but also on the playground, on field trips, or anywhere the student's same aged curriculum is expected to occur. Whereas Section I introduces the reader to what we know about PANS' impact on behavior, attention, and learning skills, Section II will describe what a careful observer might notice in these various 'classroom' settings.

Notes

---

[1] McDermott, N. (2008) New online database reveals touching tales of the first Great Ormond Street patients: http://www.dailymail.co.uk/news/article-1101696/New-online-database-reveals-touching-tales-Great-Ormond-Street-patients.html#ixzz3Uc15P5pX (retrieved, March 2015).

[2] Martino, D., Tanner, A., Defazio, G., Church, A. J, Bhatia, K. P., Giovannoni, G., Dale, R. C. (2005) Tracing Sydenham's chorea: historical documents from a British paediatric hospital. Arch Dis Child. May;90(5):507-11.

[3] English, P. C. Emergence of rheumatic fever in the nineteenth century. In Rosenberg C, Golden J, eds. Framing disease: studies in cultural history. New Brunswick, NJ: Rutgers University Press, 1991:20–32.

[4] In most cases, Impetigo results in reddish sores or blisters in the regions of the nose and mouth.

[5] The Mayo clinic describes the symptoms of Scarlet Fever as having four main symptoms: A red rash that looks like a sunburn and feels like sandpaper; red lines in the folds of skin around the groin, armpits, elbows, knees and neck; Flushed face, with a pale ring around the mouth; and a 'Strawberry' tongue, that generally looks red and bumpy, and often covered with a white coating early in the disease.(Retrieved May, 2015 from *http://www.mayoclinic.org/diseases-conditions/scarlet-fever/basics/symptoms/con-20030976*

[6] Taranta, A. & Stollerman, G. H. (1956) The relationship of Sydenham's chorea to infection with group A streptococci. The American Journal of Medicine, Volume 20, Issue 2, 170 - 175.

[7] Kirvan, C. A., Swedo, S. E., Heuser, J. S., & Cunningham, M. W. (2003) Mimicry and Auto-antibody mediated neuronal Signaling Cells in Sydenham Chorea, Nature Medicine 9, (2003) http://www.pandasnet....NMpaper[1].pdf.

[8] Still common in developing countries where resources are scarce, RHD is rarely seen in more affluent parts of the world, because of the use of antibiotics, and surgical procedures such as tonsillectomies and adenoidectomies.

[9] The American Medical Association Home Medical Encyclopedia: An A-Z Reference Guide to over 5000 Medical Terms (Vol. I and II (1989) Clayman, C.B. (Ed.) Random House NY pp 869-870.

[10] Kirvan, C. A. (2003). pp 914 - 920.

[11] Zomorrodi, A., Wald, E. R. Sydenham's chorea in western Pennsylvania. Pediatrics. 2006; 117(4):675-679.

[12] Swedo, S. E., Leonard, H.L., Schapiro, M.B., Casey, B..J., Mannheim, G.B., Lenane, M.C., Rettew, D.C. (1993) Sydenham's chorea: physical and psychological symptoms of St Vitus dance. Pediatrics. Apr 91(4):706-13.

[13] Swedo, S. E. (1994) Sydenham's Chorea: A Model for Childhood Autoimmune Neuropsychiatric Disorders *JAMA.* 1994; 272(22):1788-1791. doi:10.1001/jama.1994.03520220082035.

[14] Martino, (2005) pp 507-11.

[15] English, (1991). pp 20–32.

[16] Tanner, A. (2008) Small and special: a website of the origins of the Great Ormond Street Hospital for Children, Presentation given (GOSH) at HARG General meeting January 2008 retrieved at http://www.healtharchives.org/HARGpapers.html March 2015.

[17] Martino, (2005). pp 507-11.

[18] English, (1991). pp 20–32.

[19] Benedek, T. G. (2006). The History of Bacteriologic Concepts of Rheumatic Fever and Rheumatoid Arthritis. Semin Arthritis Rheum 36:109-123.

[20] Dr. Gene H. Stollerman is credited for his work and important 1952 publication on the usefulness of penicillin to eradicate the bacteria.

[21] The American Medical Association Home Medical Encyclopedia p 870.

[22] Swedo, S. E., Leonard, H. L., Garvey, M., Mittleman, B., Allen, A. J., Perlmutter, S., Lougee, L., Dow, S., Zamkoff, J., & Dubbert, B.K. (1998) PANDAS: Clinical Description of the First 50 Cases; Am J Psychiatry. Feb;155(2):264-71.

[23] Segen's Medical Dictionary. (2011). Retrieved March 20, 2015 from http://medical-dictionary.thefreedictionary.com/autoimmune+response.

[24] Swedo, 1998, pp 264-71.

[25] ibid.

[26] Swedo, S. E., Leonard, H. L., & Rapoport, J. L. (2004) The pediatric autoimmune neuropsychiatric disorders associated with streptococcal infection (PANDAS) subgroup: separating fact from fiction. Pediatrics:113(4):907–11.

[27] Murphy T.K., Storch, E.A., Turner, A., Reid, J. M., Tan, J., & Lewin, A. B. (2012). Clinical Factors Associated with PANDAS J Pediatr Feb; 160(2): 314–319.

[28] Swedo, (1998). pp 264-71.

[29] Swedo, S. E., Leckman, J. F., & Rose, N. R. (2012) From Research Subgroup to Clinical Syndrome Modifying the PANDAS Criteria to Describe PANS (Pediatric Acute-onset Neuropsychiatric Syndrome) Pediatrics and Therapeutics 2:113.

[30] Such as those used in Murphy, T. K., Patel, P. D., McGuire, J. F., Kennel, A., Mutch, P. J., Parker-Athill, E. C., Hanks, C. E., Lewin, A. B., Storch, E. A., Toufexi, M. D., Dadlani, G. H., & Rodriguez, C. A. (2015). Characterization of the Pediatric Acute-Onset Neuropsychiatric Syndrome Phenotype Journal of Child and Adolescent Psychopharmacology. February, 25(1): 14-25. doi:10.1089/cap.2014.0062.

[31] http://www.ncbi.nlm.nih.gov/pubmedhealth/PMH0015837/def-item/glossary.gl1-d46/

[32] There a number of ways obsessions and compulsions manifested in youth with PANS. Some may be found in Section II, along with information provided in pandasnetwork.org.

[33] Tourette's fact sheet ninds.nih, retrieved April, 2015).

[34]Information About PANDAS-NIMH website http://www.nimh.nih.gov/labs-at-nimh/research-areas/clinics-and-labs/pdnb/web.shtml, (retrieved Jan, 2015).

[35] Chang K, Frankovich, J., Cooperstock, M., Cunningham, M., Latimer, M. E., Murphy, T. K., Pasternack, M., Thienemann, M., Williams, K., Walter J., & Swedo, S. E. From the PANS Collaborative Consortium. Clinical Evaluation of Youth with Pediatric Acute-Onset Neuropsychiatric Syndrome (PANS): Recommendations from the 2013 PANS Consensus Conference Journal of Child and Adolescent Psychopharmacology. February 2015, 25(1): 3-13. doi:10.1089/cap.2014.0084.
[36] Johnson, D. R., Kurlan, R., Leckman, J., & Kaplan, E. L. The human immune response to streptococcal extracellular antigens: clinical, diagnostic, and potential pathogenetic implications. Clin Infect Dis. 2010 Feb 15;50(4):481-90. doi: 10.1086/650167.
[37] Chang, (2015). 25(1): 3-13.
[38] Murphy, (2012). pp 314–319.
[39] Regarding examples of immature bodily system, see, for example, Howard, P. (2000) The Owner's Manual for the Brain: Everyday applications from mind-brain research, 2nd edition. Austin, TX: Bard Press p 77; and immunoglobulins in all areas do not reach full maturity until adulthood or after the age of sixteen. (Jollift C.R., Karen, M., Cost, K.M., Stivrins, P.C. , Grossman, P.P., Nolte, C.R., Franco, .S.M, Fijan, K.J., Fletcher, L.L. and Shriner HC (1982) Reference Intervals for Serum IgG, IgA, 1gM,C3, and C4 as Determined by Rate Nephelometry CLIN. CHEM. 28/1, pp 126-128.)
[40] To be clear, however, there are differences in definitions between prepubertal and pediatrics. True, both terms are commonly understood to mean 'children.' However, the boundaries of the term "Pediatric Medicine" can be a bit murkier to define. Prepubertal, of course, refers to children who have not gone through puberty yet. The term 'pediatric,' however, commonly includes prepubertal children, but also adolescents. At the same time, in some jurisdictions, it may also include individuals up to the age of 18, or who are still in secondary school. In other words, "pediatric services" may be more reflective of an institution's or government's organizational and oversight operations, rather than the actual level of developmental maturity of the patient in question. Nonetheless, it is acknowledged that a host of bodily systems that are not fully developed until long after puberty (such as brain development and the immune system) are affected by this condition.
[41] Swedo, 1998, pp 264-71.
[42] Murphy, M. L., & Pichichero, M. E. (2002). Prospective identification and treatment of children with pediatric autoimmune neuropsychiatric disorder associated with group A streptococcal infection (PANDAS) Arch Pediatr Adolesc Med. 2002;156(4):356–61.
[43] Bernstein, G. A., Victor, A. M., Pipal, A. J., Williams, K. A. (2010) Comparison of clinical characteristics of pediatric autoimmune neuropsychiatric disorders associated with streptococcal infections and childhood obsessive-compulsive disorder. J Child Adolesc Psychopharmacol. Aug;20(4):333-40.
[44] Swedo, S. E., Seidlitz, J., Kovacevic, M., Latimer, M. E., Hommer, R., Lougee, L., & Grant, L. P. (2015) Journal of Child and Adolescent Psychopharmacology. February 25(1): 26-30.
[45] Swedo, (2015). pp 26-30.
[46] Swedo, (2012). 2:113.
[4747] These in turn impact classroom performance, particularly in the ability to engage and stay on task.
[48] Swedo, (2012). 2:113.
[49] Murphy, (2012). pp 314–319.
[50] Swedo, (2012). 2:113.
[51] Information About PANDAS-NIMH website http://www.nimh.nih.gov/labs-at-nimh/research-areas/clinics-and-labs/pdnb/web.shtml (retrieved Jan, 2015).
[52] Involuntary soiling of underwear with stool by youth past the age of toilet training.
[53] Swedo, (1998). 264-271.
[54] Antibodies are bodily proteins with a protective role. Often the term *antibody* is often used interchangeably with *immunoglobulin*.
[55] Kirvan, C. A., Swedo, S. E., Snider, L. A., & Cunningham M. W. (2006) Antibody-mediated neuronal cell signaling in behavior and movement disorders. J Neuroimmunol 179: 173–179 Epub 2006.
[56] Swedo S. E., & Grant, P. J. (2005): Annotation: PANDAS: a model for human autoimmune disease. J Child Psychol Psychiatry 46:227-234.
[57] Dr. Christine Kirvan is a researcher and Professor at California State University, Sacramento
[58] Kirvan, 2006, pp 173–179.
[59] Hasbi, A., O'Dowd, B. F., & George, S. R. (2011) Dopamine D1-D2 receptor heteromer signaling pathway in the brain: emerging physiological relevance. Mol Brain 4: 26.
[60] Chen, J. Y. 1, Wang, E. A., Cepeda, C., & Levine, M. S. (2013) Dopamine imbalance in Huntington's disease: a mechanism for the lack of behavioral flexibility. Front Neurosci. Jul 4;7:114. doi: 10.3389/fnins.2013.00114. eCollection 2013.
[61] Sweeney, M. S. (2009) Brain: The Complete Mind: how it Develops, how it Works, and how to Keep it Sharp. National Geographic Books, Washington, DC p 151.
[62] Chen, (2013), Jul 4; 7:114.
[63] Sweeney. (2009), pp 52-53.
[64] Morgan, (2005) The Midbrain (Gray Matter) Chelsea House Publications, Philadelphia. pp 24-27.
[65] (Sometimes antibodies are used interchangeably with immunoglobulins).
[66] Kirvan, (2006), pp 173–179.
[67] Kirvan, C.A., Cox, C. J., Swedo, S. E., & Cunningham, M.W. (2007) Tubulin is a neuronal target of autoantibodies in Sydenham's chorea. J Immunol. Jun 1;178(11):7412-21.
[68] Brimberg, L., Benhar, I., Mascaro-Blanco, A., Alvarez, K., Lotan, D., Winter, C., Klein, J., Moses, A. E., Somnier, F. E., Leckman, J. F., Swedo, S. E., Cunningham, M. W., & Joel, D. (2012) Behavioral, Pharmacological, and Immunological Abnormalities after Streptococcal Exposure: A Novel Rat Model of Sydenham Chorea and Related Neuropsychiatric Disorders. Neuropsychopharmacology. Aug;37(9):2076-87. doi: 10.1038/npp.2012.56. Epub 2012 Apr 25.

[69] Ben-Pazi, H., Stoner, J. A., & Cunningham, M. W. (2013). Dopamine Receptor Autoantibodies Correlate with Symptoms in Sydenham's Chorea. PLoS ONE, 8(9), e73516. doi:10.1371/journal.pone.0073516.
[70] Cox, C. J., Sharma, M., Leckman, J. F., Zuccolo, J., Zuccolo, A., Kovoor, Swedo S. E., Cunningham, M. W. (2013). Brain Human Monoclonal Autoantibody from Sydenham Chorea Targets Dopaminergic Neurons in Transgenic Mice and Signals Dopamine D2 Receptor: Implications in Human Disease. Journal of Immunology (Baltimore, Md. : 1950), 191(11), 10.4049/jimmunol.1102592. doi:10.4049/jimmunol.1102592.
[71] Ben-Pazi, 2013, PLoS ONE, 8(9).
[72] Kirvan, C. A., Swedo, S. E., Snider, L. A., & Cunningham, M. W. (2006) Antibody-mediated neuronal cell signaling in behavior and movement disorders. J Neuroimmunol 179: 173–179 Epub 2006.
[73] Candelaria Greene, JF (2015) Unpublished survey of family members, providers, and survivors of PANS regarding PANS and Education (2013-2015), collected as UC Berkeley Visiting Researcher Scholar, Berkeley, California.
[74] Thamotharampillai, D., Smith, D., Knowland, D., Hsu, M., Platt, M., Bittner-Eddy, P., Cohen, B., Southern, P., Latimer, E., Harley, E., Dritan Agalliu, D., & Cleary, P. P. (2016) Group A Streptococcus intranasal infection promotes CNS infiltration by streptococcal-specific Th17 cells. J Clin Invest. 2016;126(1):303-317. (Originally published 12/14/2015).
[75] Columbia University Medical Center (CUMC) Newsroom: How Recurrent Strep A Infections Affect the Brain: Newly discovered route by which immune cells reach the brain may underlie an autoimmune neuropsychiatric disorder in children. http://newsroom.cumc.columbia.edu/blog/2015/12/15/strepabrain/.
[76] Also see the excellent youtube.com video where Doctors Cleary and Agalliu elegantly explain their findings. (https://www.youtube.com/watch?v=HlpzWGS6f60).
[77] An axon is part of a neuron. Its function is to send information to different neurons, muscles and glands.
[78] CUMC Newsroom 12/15/15.
[79] Singer, H. S., Gilbert, D. L., Wolf, D. S., Mink, J. W., Kurlan, R. (2012) Moving from PANDAS to CANS.J Pediatr. 2012 May;160(5):725-31. doi: 10.1016/j.jpeds.2011.11.040. Epub 2011 Dec 22.
[80] Swedo, 2012, 2:113.
[81] ibid.
[82] Chang, (2015). 25(1): 3-13.
[83] Swedo, (2012). 2:113.
[84] Chang, (2015). 25(1): 3-13.
[85] ibid.
[86] ibid.
[87] Frankovich, J., Thienemann, M., Pearlstein, J., Crable, A., Brown, K., & Chang, K. (2015) Multidisciplinary clinic dedicated to treating youth with pediatric acute-onset neuropsychiatric syndrome: presenting characteristics of the first 47 consecutive patients. J Child Adolesc Psychopharmacol. 2015 Feb;25(1):38-47. doi: 10.1089/cap.2014.0081.
[88] Murphy, M. L.,& Pichichero, M. E. (2002). Prospective identification and treatment of children with pediatric autoimmune neuropsychiatric disorder associated with group A streptococcal infection (PANDAS) Arch Pediatr Adolesc Med. 2002;156(4):356–61. [PubMed].
[89] Snider, L. A., Lougee, L., Slattery, M., Grant, P., & Swedo, S. E. (2005) Antibiotic prophylaxis with azithromycin or penicillin for childhood-onset neuropsychiatric disorders. Biol Psychiatry. 57(7):788-92.
[90] Kovacevic, M., Grant, P., & Swedo, S. E. (2015) Journal of Child and Adolescent Psychopharmacology. February 2015, 25(1): 65-69. doi:10.1089/cap.2014.0067.
[91] Perlmutter, S. J., Leitman, S. F., Garvey, M. A., Hamburger, S., Feldman, E., Leonard, H. L., & Swedo, S. E. (1999): Therapeutic plasma exchange and intravenous immunoglobulin for obsessive-compulsive disorder and tic disorders in childhood. Lancet 1999, 354:1153-1158.
[92] Latimer, M. E., L'Etoile, N., Seidlitz, J., & Swedo, S. E. (2015) J Child Adolesc Psychopharmacol. Therapeutic plasma apheresis as a treatment for 35 severely ill children and adolescents with pediatric autoimmune neuropsychiatric disorders associated with streptococcal infections.Feb;25(1):70-5. doi: 10.1089/cap.2014.0080. Epub 2015 Feb 6.
[93] Perlmutter, S. J., Leitman, S. F., Garvey, M. A., Hamburger, S., Feldman, E., Leonard, H. L., & Swedo, S. E. (1999): Therapeutic plasma exchange and intravenous immunoglobulin for obsessive-compulsive disorder and tic disorders in childhood. Lancet 1999, 354:1153-1158.
[94] Information About PANDAS-NIMH website http://www.nimh.nih.gov/labs-at-nimh/research-areas/clinics-and-labs/pdnb/web.shtml, (retrieved Jan, 2015).
[95] Swedo, (2012). 2:113.
[96] Murphy, T. K., Storch, E. A., & Strawser, M. S. (2006) Selective serotonin reuptake inhibitor-induce behavioral activation in the PANDAS subtype, Primary Psychiatry; 13(8):87-89.
[97] Swedo, (2012). 2:113.
[98] Storch, E. A., Murphy, T. K., Geffken, G. R., Mann, G., Adkins, J., Merlo, L. .J., Duke, D., Munson, M., Swaine, Z., & Goodman, W. K. (2006) Cognitive-behavioral therapy for PANDAS-related obsessive-compulsive disorder: Findings from a preliminary waitlist controlled open trial. J Am Acad Child Adolesc Psychiatry. 2006 Oct;45(10):1171-8.
[99] Candelaria Greene. (2015), Unpublished Survey (2013-2015).
[100] *pandasnetwork.org* PANDAS/PANS Statistics 2014-2015http://pandasnetwork.org/wp-content/uploads/2014/11/Statistics-PANDAS-Network.pdf (retrieved April 2015).
[101] Swedo, (1998). pp 264-71.
[102] *pandasnetwork.org* , 2015 PANDAS/PANS Statistics 2014-2015).
[103] Swedo, (1998). pp 264-71.
[104] National Diabetes Statistics Report, 2014 www.diabetes.org National Federation for the Blind https://nfb.org/blindness-statistics Retrieved April 2015.

[105] American Printing House for the Blind, "Annual Report 2014: Distribution of Eligible Students Based on the Federal Quota Census of January 7, 2013 (Fiscal Year 2014)." Accessed July 28, 2014, from http://www.aph.org/federal-quota/dist14.html.
[106] American Cancer Society Cancer Facts and Figures, 2014 (Retrieved April 1, 2005) http://www.cancer.org/research/cancerfactsstatistics/cancerfactsfigures2014/.
[107] "Low incidence" is a term used in US Education/ Special Education to mean disabling conditions that affect a very small percentage of students requiring special education or other services.
[108] Candelaria Greene, J. F. (2015). Unpublished Survey (2013-2015).
[109] ibid. When most people think of students who receive special help or accommodations in schools, they usually think of students with learning disabilities. Interestingly, however, none of these students ever qualified for services under *'specific learning disability,'* which would have been identified through formal testing at the schools (or privately in the community). What this means is that in these cases, either the student's skills were "too high," (even with the debilitating symptoms of PANS) to qualify under a 'specific learning disability' and/***or*** the family and school simply addressed student needs based on the *medical* or *psychiatric* condition (that the families sought out for themselves and presented to the schools).
[110] ibid. These students also reported that they had at least one school staff member who was going to 'make it happen' for them, no matter what it took.
[111] Pavone, P., Bianchini, R., Parano, E., Incorpora, G., Rizzo, R., Mazzone, L., & Trafiletti, R. R.: Anti-brain antibodies in PANDAS versus uncomplicated streptococcal infection. Pediatr Neurol 2004, 30:107-10.
[112] Kumar, A., Williams, M., Muzik, O. and Chugani, H. (2014) Basal ganglia inflammation in children with neuropsychiatric symptoms J Nucl Med. 2014; 55 (Supplement 1):306.
[113] Sweeney, M. S. (2009) Brain: The Complete Mind: how it Develops, how it Works, and how to Keep it Sharp. National Geographic Books, Washington, DC. p 309.
[114] Morgan, M. (2005) The Midbrain (Gray Matter) Chelsea House Publications, Philadelphia. p 27.
[115] Chakravarthy V. S., Joseph, D., & Bapi, R. S. (2010) Biol Cybern. What do the basal ganglia do? A modeling perspective.Sep;103(3):237-53. doi: 10.1007/s00422-010-0401-y. Epub 2010 Jul 20.
[116] Howard, P. (2000) The Owner's Manual for the Brain: Everyday applications from mind-brain research, 2nd edition. Austin, TX: Bard Press p 389.
[117] As reported by researchers Dr. Dritan Agalliu and Dr. Patrick Cleary. (Thamotharampillai, Smith, and Knowland et al. (2016).
[118] Sweeney, (2009). p 161.
[119] Morgan, (2005). p 27.
[120] Morgan, (2005). p28.
[121] Chakravarthy, (2010). pp 237-53.
[122] Bear, M. F., Connors, B. W. & Paradiso, M. A., Neuroscience: Exploring the Brain, Second Edition, Lippincott Williams & Wilkins, 2001, pp 473-482.
[123] Purves, D., Augustine, G. J., & Fitzpatrick, D., et al., editors. (2001) Neuroscience. 2nd edition. Sunderland (MA): Sinauer Associates. Projections from the Basal Ganglia to Other Brain Regions. Available from: http://www.ncbi.nlm.nih.gov/books/NBK10860/.
[124] Herrero, M. T. 1, Barcia, C., Navarro, J. M. (2002) Functional anatomy of thalamus and basal ganglia. Childs Nerv Syst. Aug;18(8):386-404. Epub 2002 Jul 26.
[125] Booth, J. R., Wood, L., Lu, D., Houk, J.C., & Bitan, T. (2007) The role of the basal ganglia and cerebellum in language processing. Brain Research. 1133:136–44.
[126] Bear, M. F., Connors, B. W., & Paradiso, M. A. (2001).
[127] Hikosaka, O. (1989) Role of basal ganglia in saccades. Rev Neurol (Paris). 145(8-9):580-6.
[128] Herrero, M. T., Barcia, C., Navarro, J. M. (2002) Functional anatomy of thalamus and basal ganglia. Childs Nerv Syst. Aug;18(8):386-404. Epub 2002 Jul 26.
[129] Pederson, R. A. & Troost, B. T. (1981) Stroke Abnormalities of Gaze in Cerebrovascular Disease in Current Concepts of Cerebrovascular Disease. Stroke, Vol 12, No 2, 1981.
[130] Findlay, J. M. & Gilchrist, I. D. (2003) Active vision: the psychology of looking and seeing. Oxford; New York: Oxford University Press, Series: Oxford psychology series, no. 37.
[131] Ings, S (2008). A natural history of seeing: the art and science of vision. PP 17-18, 44-47 Publisher: New York: W.W. Norton, p.18.
[132] Starr, M. S., & Rayner, K. (2001) Eye movements during reading: some current controversies TRENDS in Cognitive Sciences Vol.5 No.4 April 2001.
[133] Pederson, (1981).
[134] Morgan, (2006). p 102.
[135] Booth, (2007). pp 136-44.
[136] Delazer, M., Domahs, F., Lochy, A., Karner, E., Benke, T., & Poewe, W. (2003) Number processing and basal ganglia dysfunction: a single case study Neuropsychologia Volume 42, Issue 8, 2004, pp 1050–1062.
[137] Murphy, T. K., Patel, P. D., McGuire, J. F., Kennel, A., Mutch, P. J., Parker-Athill, E. C., Hanks, C. E., Lewin, A. B., Storch, E. A., Toufexi, M. D., Dadlani, G. H., and &, C. A. (2015). Characterization of the Pediatric Acute-Onset Neuropsychiatric Syndrome Phenotype Journal of Child and Adolescent Psychopharmacology. February 2015, 25(1): 14-25. doi:10.1089/cap.2014.0062.
[138] Lewin, A. B., Storch, E. A., Mutch, P. J., & Murphy, T. K. Neurocognitive functioning in youth with pediatric autoimmune neuropsychiatric disorders associated with streptococcus. J Neuropsychiatry Clin Neurosci. 2011 Fall;23(4):391-8. doi: 10.1176/appi.neuropsych.23.4.391.
[139] Hirschtritt, M. E., Hammond, C. J., Luckenbaugh, D., Buhle, J., Thurm, A. E., Casey, B. J., & Swedo, S. E. Executive and attention functioning among children in the PANDAS subgroup (2009) Child Neuropsychol. Mar;15(2):179-94. Epub 2008 Jul 11.

[140] Sweeney, (2009). pp 86-87.
[141] ibid.
[142] Intermittent eye dilation is often a prominent physical symptom of amygdala dysfunction.
[143] As noted in numerous participants' comments (Candelaria Greene, 2015. Unpublished Survey (2013-2015).
[144] Research on this topic is in development, specifically that of pediatric neurologist and research Dr. Beth Latimer, which may show whether strep, staph, or other bacteria is hiding in the tonsillar crypts, as noted by pandasnetwork.org. (From http://pandasnetwork.org/jama-case-report-tonsillectomy-in-pandas-treatment/Jan 13, 201).
[145] Cunningham, M. W. (2009). Molecular Mimicry; Published Online: 15 SEP 2009
DOI: 10.1002/9780470015902.a0000958.pub2 2001 John Wiley & Sons, Ltd.
[146] Kirvan, C. A., Swedo, S. E., Heuser, J. S., & Cunningham, M. W. (2003) Mimicry and Auto-antibody mediated neuronal Signaling Cells in Sydenham Chorea, Nature Medicine 9, 914 - 920 http://www.pandasnet....NMpaper[1].pdf
[147] ibid.
[148] Pavone, P., Bianchini, R., Parano, E., Incorpora, G., Rizzo, R., Mazzone, L., & Trafiletti, R. R. (2004): Anti-brain antibodies in PANDAS versus uncomplicated streptococcal infection. Pediatr Neurol 2004 30:107-10.
[149] Kirvan, 2003, pp 914-920.
[150] The converse is also true. As access to appropriate medical care improves for these youth, identification and incidence levels will most likely reflect what are assumed levels.
[151] Murphy,(2015). 14-25.
[152] ibid.
[153] As reported by participants surveyed (Candelaria Greene, 2015. Unpublished Survey (2013-2015).
[154] Diana Pohlman is the founder and Executive Director Emeritus of PANDASnetwork.org, an advocacy organization devoted to the cause of helping families of youth with PANDAS/PANS.
[155] The noted author of "Saving Sammy," Beth Maloney opened many parents' eyes to the possibility that their children too, (who were suffering similar symptoms) might actually be suffering from PANDAS.
[156] As used in the work of Dr. J. Frankovich (Frankovich, 2015, pp 38-47).

Section II

SPECIFIC BEHAVIORAL AND COGNITIVE ASPECTS OF PANS:

What the Careful Observer May Notice

What differences in behavior, learning, and attention can be seen in students affected by PANS? As clearly as the symptomatology for PANS is laid out in its diagnostic criteria, one can still expect to see a wide variation in its expression. The depth and breadth of symptoms will be exacerbated, or limited, by a number of factors, including how long the individual has had the condition before receiving treatment, the age of onset, and the number of repeated exposures and exacerbations. Moreover, as a greater exposure to such triggering agents as harmful bacterias and viruses can occur during the winter months, one can therefore expect to see an increase in PANS-related symptoms during the 'cold and flu season.' Other contributing factors include the student's quality of sleep, nutritional intake and assimilation, and symptomatic relief (or exacerbation) resulting from various therapeutic treatment modalities. The important thing to keep in mind is that, as with any other broad-reaching illness, PANS has no *one-size-fits-all* presentation.

For some students, PANS can represent an extended period of serious debilitation across functional domains and lines of development. At the same time, for others, especially if the illness is treated promptly, it may constitute a mere 'blip' on their medical and educational radar screens towards adulthood.

The following presents an overview of some behaviors and characteristics that may be linked to PANS symptomatology. Following this review, we then draw back the lens to take a 'macro view,' of how certain types of functioning require multiple skills and processing abilities to carry out smoothly. In taking a closer look at the multifaceted demands that are required for language skills and executive function, for example, one can easily grasp how efficiency in either area can be thwarted by its weakest component. Moreover, we can understand how such multifaceted skills can, in turn, affect the development of other abilities, such as that needed for the formation of a *critical perspective* (or considered and thoughtful point of view).

In looking at the following overview, it is very important that the reader be cognizant of three important caveats. First, *most of these behaviors and characteristics can be observed, to some degree, at different junctures in most students' academic experience.* What separates what is considered to be 'within normal parameters' and 'PANS behaviors,' is often the *jagged and substantial degree in which a breadth of domains is affected*. Secondly, identifying the **frequency** and **duration** of symptoms will be key. The specific symptoms (OCD, tic, etc), should be noted, but also their frequency throughout the day, and how, or if, they alter over time. This second caveat is important because one parent or staff member's *interpretation of the same behavior* will vary from another's.[1] Moreover, one parent's subjective opinion of **severity of symptoms** can differ from another parent's. Ultimately though, *any* student exhibiting a cluster of the following behaviors should be referred to the appropriate provider for follow up, as clusters can signal indications of PANS (or other conditions) that should be diagnosed or ruled out. Thirdly, this list is, by no means exhaustive. It is merely *a sampling of behaviors* noted in PANS literature and reported by parents, PANS survivors, providers, and others.[2]

Finally, we shift the lens away from the classroom and focus on the family. Schools and students do not, and cannot, operate in a vacuum. The critical interdependence of the student/school/family triad quickly becomes apparent when an illness as debilitating as PANS strikes. For those students whose PANS' symptoms *do not* represent a transient blip of childhood illnesses, the extent to which functioning can occur in an academic environment (or any other environment, for that matter) will largely depend on the levels and types of assistance he receives at home.

That said, the extraordinary levels of support that are needed to continually bolster this child come at a cost-financially, physically, and emotionally. With this in mind, it behooves the observer to be aware of changes that one might notice among family members during the PANS journey as well, and examples of these are presented at the end of this section.

Observable Changes in the School Setting

As we shall see in Section III, in order for academic learning to progress, a student's medical and psychological well-being has first got to be addressed, or at the very least, *stabilized*. As readers peruse the following list of 'observable changes in the school setting,' they are strongly advised to consider them as ***symptoms of a medical illness***. This becomes essential later on, as teams gather to consider those interventions and modifications that will not only support the student, but reduce further exacerbations of their symptoms.

1. Appearance

Staff and others may notice the following:

- Increased Absenteeism. The most obvious thing that one may notice among students affected by PANS is their *absence*. A *decrease* in attendance and an *increase* in tardiness may be due to a combination of factors, such as attendance at medical or other appointments, lethargy from having had had a poor night's sleep the night before, weakened ability to organize themselves to be prepared for school on time, or **separation anxiety** surrounding leaving their home or their parent. Increased absenteeism can also stem from the student's own sense of school failure and underachievement, whereby in a desperate effort to avoid repeated failure and humiliation, he refuses to attend school altogether. Moreover, school refusal can result from sensory (or any other type of) overwhelm, whereby the student feels that he can no longer risk participation in that environment.
- Changes in Posture. This may be related to issues related to health, fitness, or psychological factors. Hypotonia, or floppy posture, has also been reported.[3]
- Poor Skin Color. This can be possibly related to the illness, and/or to decreased amounts of time spent outside, etc.
- Look of Tiredness. This may be secondary to decreased amounts of sleep, changes in mood or anxiety, and to symptoms of the illness (such as those associated with increased cytokines[4] that facilitate the production of sleep producing histamines). (*Excessive sleepiness during the day* may be also indicative of other serious medical conditions. In any case, medical attention should be sought out immediately.)
- Reduced Neatness in the Student's Work Area or Desk. This can be due to a number of factors, including worsening fine motor skills, poorer memory, and the increased need for time to complete the same activity.
- Poor Grooming. Again, this can be due to weakened fine motor and attentional skills, poorer awareness of how they are presenting themselves, or worsening time management. Also OCD (Obsessive Compulsive Disorder) triggers are acknowledged to have a 'nesting nature,' presenting as perfectionism, or fixation on activities that are performed at home. As a result, successful or thorough completion of self-care activities are either prevented or delayed.
- Evidence of Skin Picking.
- More Cuts and Scrapes. This may be possibly due to self-harm.
- Bald Spots and Thinning Hair. This may be due to hair pulling or Trichotillomania.
- Poor Eye Contact. This may be secondary to changes in mood, visual perception, or even difficulties in being able to process auditory and visual information simultaneously.
- Hyperventilation (or taking deep breaths, without apparent asthma). This can be illness related.
- Dilated Pupils. This is a common indicator found among students affected by PANS.[5]

- More Active (or Fidgety) than Usual, Hyperactive. This may be secondary to weakening body awareness (proprioception), the need to move about to stay awake, or other factors related to the illness.
- Keeping to Oneself. One may observe less interaction with peers, as social relationships and participation in playground games become increasingly difficult to maintain.

2. Simple and Complex Tics

These may include:

- Vocal Tics (i.e.) repetitive sniffing, coughs, cries, barking sounds, or words.
- Unexpected Voice Changes.
- Unexpected Movements that can include head jerking or constant blinking.

Secondary symptoms or related phenomena may include:

- Increased Requests to Go to the Bathroom. May use the bathroom as a place of respite; may also use bathroom during class time as a *safe time* to use facilities, or to just move about and let off energy. At the same time, urinary frequency is a component of the physical neuronal process having to do with serotonin dysregulation.[6] (Children do not feel they have voided and/or they have a feeling of wetness).
- Increased Isolation from Peers in attempts to hide uncontrolled movements or sounds.
- Quizzical Looks and Comments from Peers surrounding student's movements or sounds.

Note: See also examples of tics (from the *YGTSS*) in the appendices.

3. Other Unexpected Movements

These may include the following:

- Hyperventilation
- Inability to Sustain a Steady Grip on Items Such as Writing or Eating Utensils. In some instances, this may include what is called a "milk maid grasp."
- Increase in Behaviors Commonly Associated with Hyperactivity.
- Unexpected Head Jerking.
- Constant or Atypical Blinking.
- Complex Coughs which can include, for example, tapping, or hitting wall.
- Flailing Arm.

Secondary symptoms or related phenomena may include:

- Increased Requests to Go to the Bathroom. (May be used as a respite from peers as tics worsen).

4. Mood Changes and Anxiety

Indications of mood changes and anxiety can include:

- Changes in Concentration, Decisiveness, and Attention.
- Excessive Crying and Laughing, Rapid or Slowed Speech, Heightened or Lowered Levels of Activity, and Other Types of Mood Lability. (May be associated with the illness itself or changes/side effects of prescribed medications).
- Behaviors Described as "Panic Attacks" (such as pressure in chest or chest pain, or heart pounding very fast).
- More Reactive to Sensory Overwhelm than Before (from lights, sounds, etc.).

Secondary symptoms or related phenomena may include:

- Poor Eye Contact stemming from reduced levels with, and by, peers and others.
- Increased Isolation From Peers. Also, does not appear to seek out interactions with peers as before.
- Lack of Stamina in doing activities that were once enthusiastically engaged in.
- Reduction in School Work Projects and Homework.
- Appears Tired, Constantly Looks away from Activity, Looks Preoccupied (possibly due to overwhelm worry, or fatigue).
- Complains (or Shows Indication of) Stomach Ache or of Other Somatic Condition.
- More Sensitive and Reactive to Peers' Comments and Behaviors than Before. Behaviors can display as more emotional, crying, and self-deprecating, (or) more reactive, confrontational, or agitated. May negatively or wrongly interpret, under-assess, and devalue others actions and words, as well as their own.[7]
- Physical and Verbal Aggression as a response to lowered frustration tolerances or increased impulsivity.
- Weaker Quality and Quantity of Peer Relationships. Relationships may become more one sided. May not have the energy or enthusiasm to 'put out' enough energy to maintain conversations, interactions, and activities, as before.
- More Reactive to Changes in Class Routine. May regress and be less functional if the teacher removes student supports (such as a daily posting of the schedule for the day on the class overhead, etc.).

Note:

- ➢ Note that many of the observable behaviors that are listed in other areas of this section can be traced to, and will overlap with, changes in mood and anxiety.
- ➢ Especially with regard to mood and anxiety symptoms, it is important that schools be made aware of any related medications that the student is taking, in that sometimes these can exacerbate PANS symptoms further. The school can provide critical data points in this regard, as they can help to gauge the effectiveness and possible side-effects of such medications during school hours.

5. Emotional and Social Regression to One Much Younger

- May Demonstrate a Regression in Coping Skills, Social Awareness, or Social Language Skills. May be more noticeable amongst peers than with (one on one) interactions with adults.

6. Obsessive Compulsive Disorder (OCD)

- The DSM V describes *Obsessions* as *"recurrent and persistent thoughts, urges, or images that are experienced as intrusive and unwanted."*[8] Examples of obsessions include Fixations, Scrupulosity, or Perfectionism (such as rewriting papers, etc.).
- *Compulsions* are described as *"repetitive behaviors or mental acts that an individual feels driven to perform in response to an obsession or according to rules that must be applied rigidly".*[9] Examples of compulsions include counting, tapping, reassurances of various sorts, spitting, etc.
- The DSM V notes that *"some other obsessive-compulsive and related disorders are also characterized by preoccupations and by repetitive behaviors or mental acts in response to the preoccupation,"* while others *"are characterized primarily by recurrent body-focused repetitive behaviors (e.g. hair pulling, skin picking) and repeated attempts to decrease or stop the behaviors."*[10]
- There are as many variations of OCD as there are personality types. See also examples of obsessions and compulsions taken from the CY-BOCS (in appendices).

The following may be indicative of behaviors stemming from OCD:

- Lateness or Absence from School because of extended morning routines (i.e. 20 minutes to sterilize comb from contamination concerns; the lengthily *'tooth brushing ceremony'* which surrounds a time consuming ritual of oral health care, etc.).
- Spitting at Inappropriate Times or Places.
- Shutting Cupboards or Drawers "the correct way," after others have closed them.
- Unexpected Fears, Concerns, or Questions (such as questions surrounding the health or whereabouts of others, or the expiration dates of foods).
- Changes in Appropriate Conversational 'Turn Taking.' The student may repeat questions to determine 'certainty.' He wants 'exact' answers; appears to view responses as 'black or white.' He may need to feel responses are 'just right.'
- Reduction in Capacity for Awareness (or Perceived Concern) of How Others Are Seeing Him.
- Subtle or Overt Types of 'Accommodating Behaviors' (such as that which follows below).
- Uses More Facial Tissue than otherwise Expected (Without Obvious Nasal Congestion). This may be a possible compensatory behavior to disguise or accommodate for issues surrounding saliva (or fears of contamination/germs).
- Exhibits Repetitive Behaviors (including counting, or repeating words or actions).
- Needs More Time/Slower Transitions (due to accommodating behaviors).
- Oddnesses In Speech- (May also result from need to pool saliva or the need to say things in a **particular manner**.)
- Noted Differences In Behaviors At School From What Is Reported At Home. Family may see more behaviors due to 'nesting' nature of OCD.[11] [12]
- Excessive Use of Erasers.
- Appearing to Need to Have Everything 'Perfect.'

- Changes in Eating Habits, such as separating foods on plate so that the foods do not touch each other, or suddenly becoming a very 'picky' eater.

For some students with PANS, the sheer intensity and profound discomfort of the OCD- as with intense overwhelm from mood, anxiety, or other stressors- may result in extreme reactivity, that for the onlooker, would interpret as being not only serious, but in some cases, aggressive and harmful, and that require immediate communication and interventions from parents, staff, and appropriate professionals.

A few examples include:

- Restrictive Eating to the Point of Not Eating.
- Screaming and Other Verbal Outbursts.
- Tantrums That Come on Easily and that Can Last a Long Time (sometimes days.)
- Hitting Walls or Other Structures in Response to Specific or Unknown Stressors.
- Running Away From Parents or School Staff.
- Language Stating that They "Want to Die." *(Such language may stem from the intense discomfort of the symptoms that this student may be feeling. At the same time, any such language or behavior that indicates potential harm to self or others warrants immediate communication and intervention from appropriate parties.)*
- Pulling Out Hair (i.e. Trichotillomania).
- Initiating Physical or Verbal Contact with Others in Potentially Harmful Ways.
- Engaging In Behaviors that Physically Harms Self, (such as repeatedly striking their hand against a structure or themselves, or head banging).
- Refusing To Get Into Cars, and Threats and/or Attempts to Jump Out of Cars.
- Exhibiting the Need to 'Control' Parents and Others Verbal Responses, Health, and Location.
- Excessive Touching of People, Items, or Self.
- A 'Hyper focus' on the OCD Thought, at the Expense of the Student's Own Safety or Concern for Current Circumstances.

Moreover, some PANS-stricken students *may appear* oppositional or defiant to those in authority. Perhaps they may have even been diagnosed as having Oppositional Defiant Disorder (ODD). Some examples of such behavior include:

- Not Stopping an Activity When Told to Do So.
- Hitting or Pushing Individuals Who Attempt to Control Them.
- Refusing to Carry Out Instructions of Those in Authority.
- Screaming, or Verbal Abusing Individuals in Authoritative Positions.
- Disobeying Commonly Acknowledged Rules of School.

Note:

- Sometimes, it may be extremely difficult to distinguish OCD symptoms from sensory overload issues. Some behaviors may be learned accommodations for heightened tactile, auditory, visual, or olfactory overloads.[13]
- The above list includes only a few of the many variations of OCD as they might present in a school setting. As OCD is a major component of PANS, educators and others are advised to seek out additional resources in this regard.

- Of course, the behaviors listed above underlie the critical importance of working with a qualified psychologist who is knowledgeable about PANS-related symptoms regarding the educational planning and care of this student.

7. Executive Function

- Aspects of Executive Function include attentional skills, predicting, planning, and organization. Moreover, **working memory** and language are essential components in executive function, as is impulse control.
- Difficulties in this area often overlap with symptoms of ADHD as well.
- Associated with the regulation of attention, emotion, and social functioning.[14]

Indications of possible dysfunction in this area include:

- Increased Incidence of Tardiness.
- Forgetfulness of Tasks that are Needed for Homework.
- Worsened Time Management.
- Completed Homework that is not brought to School.
- Completed Work brought to School, but not Turned in on Time, or to the Right Person/Area.
- Poor Eye Contact with listener/speaker or with task at hand.
- High Distractibility.
- Poor Task Completion (especially on tasks that require multiple steps).
- Poor Planning and Organization of Written Work and Projects.
- Messy Backpack, Locker, and Working Areas.
- Constantly Losing Things.
- Poorer Grooming. Shoes are loosely tied or go untied altogether. Shoes themselves may not be put on completely. In males, zippers may not be fully zipped.
- Transitions Take a Longer Time. May (need to be) the last to arrive and the last to leave class.
- Poor Sense of Sequencing *"First, Next, Last."*
- Markedly Reduced Ability to 'Multitask.' For example, the student may no longer be able to listen to the instructor, write lecture notes, and comprehend material simultaneously.

Note:

- Certain medications (i.e. methylphenidate) used to treat ADHD can sometimes be associated with visual processing difficulties (blurred vision, visual hallucinations). It is important that the school be informed of the medications that the student is taking, in order to provide feedback.
- Behaviors attributed to poor executive function might be secondary to poor auditory signaling, weakened visual processing ability, or lethargy or attentional difficulties associated with the illness itself.

8. Visual Processing

- Aspects of Visual Processing include (visual) attention, memory, binocular vision (having to do with both eyes working together efficiently), tracking, visual closure, and processing speed.
- In a study of youth with PANDAS, a marked *impairment in visuospatial memory* was associated with Group A beta-hemolytic Streptococcus titer elevations.[15]

- In this same study by Dr. Lewin and colleagues, a marked *impairment in visuospatial recall memory* was also observed. This, in spite of average to above-average performance on academic and other neurocognitive measures.[16]

Students with visual processing difficulties may:

- Require Much Longer to Read Text and Numbers.
- Require Much Longer to Complete Tasks, especially if these require visual processing *and* fine motor skills (such as writing).
- Appear to Have Dilated Pupils (which can also be associated with an increased sensitivity to light sources, and may result in the need for reduced screen time or sunglasses, etc).[17]
- Struggle with Encoding, Remembering, and Using Visual Information when it is Simultaneously Presented with Auditory, Kinesthetic, or Other Sensory Information. However, this student may continue to make sense of, and be able to process, visual information when looking at *singular images*, (such as a stationary chess board, or a photograph).*
- Demonstrate Difficulty with Reading Body Language and Facial Cues.
- Demonstrate Difficulties with Word Tracking in Books, Movie Subtitles, etc. Weaknesses in word tracking can, in turn, affect reading rate and comprehension.
- Display Changes in Eye Contact with Others (possibly stemming from an inability to process auditory and visual information at the same time).
- Cannot Take Notes and Listen to Lectures at the Same Time, especially if it is of 'low interest.'
- (More than his Peers), Seem Exhausted, Overwhelmed, or 'Tuned out' after Short Periods of Work that Require Visual Attention, Processing, and Sustained Mental Effort.
- Demonstrate Difficulties in Remembering *Rapid Sequences of Visual Information.* In contrast with his same aged peers, he or she may not be able to remember, understand, or synthesize segments of movies, videos, actions of others, or sites viewed from a moving vehicle.
- Show Marked Changes in Handwriting (clarity, size, slant, etc). Changes in motor planning when working across the page; cannot write in a straight line.
- Have Difficulty with Copying, or Does Not Copy, from Blackboard or Overhead.
- Have Increased Number of Math Errors Due to "Oversight."
- Demonstrate an Increase in Math Errors (reversing "+" and "–" on number lines, quadrant labeling, transferring work to graphs.
- Do not do Crossword Puzzles (and other Similar 'Fun' Activities), or Take a Very Long Time to Complete.
- Get Lost or Needs Extra Monitoring/ Guidance on Field Trips, especially if walking is required.
- Are Slower in Transitions. He or she is slower in going from activity to activity, topic to topic, and place to place. (Last one to get there- last one to leave).
- Keep Messy, Disorganized Backpacks, and have difficulty retrieving items they may (or may not) have placed there.
- Lose Homework, Supplies, Pencils, etc.
- Lose Place When Tracking Text.
- Demonstrate Poor Organizational Skills.
- Look Poorly Groomed/Weakened Grooming Skills.

Note:

- Weakened visual processing affects other skill areas, including fine motor, gross motor, and memory skills.
- *As Dr. Mark Anderson of UC Berkeley School of Optometry notes, *three dimensional images*, such as human movement and body language observed in real-life day-to-day exchanges, require the processing of *far more 'data points,' and energy,* than if that same individual were watching a *two dimensional image*, such as a computer screen. It is no wonder then, that PANS-affected families often report that their student can maintain the ability to navigate computer programs, even while suffering from other symptoms of the illness.[18]

9. Auditory Processing Changes

Indications of difficulties in this area can include:

- Poor Follow-Through on Verbal Directions.
- Weakened Auditory Memory *Sequencing* (First, next, last) of the *what, where, who,* and *why.*
- Poor Memory of the *Details* of Spoken Language, music (including lyrics), or other collections of sounds.
- Poor Sound to Letter (Phonics) Awareness (more likely to be observed in the primary grades).
- Looking Out the Window.
- Poor Interpretation, or Recall, of Oral Presentations by Teachers, etc.
- Missed Steps in Math and other work that was previously explained.
- Increased Difficulty with Processing Spoken Language. (May now make more requests that verbal instructions are repeated.)
- Increased Difficulty in Formulating Language. He or she is less quick, spontaneous, and verbal than before, and less conversant.
- Less Fluency in Carrying Out Tasks that Require Language and Fine Motor Ability (such as listening and note-taking).

Note:

- Extreme sensitivity to sound can indicate overstimulation of auditory receptors, which can result in sensory overwhelm. Care must be taken to allow the student to express his need for a quieter environment.
- May be secondary to ear, nose, and throat inflammation from infections or allergies, which in turn, can lead to poor auditory signaling.
- Symptoms may also be secondary to poor executive function.

10. Gross Motor Skills

Students who struggle in this area may:

- Lose Energy.
- Demonstrate Increased Clumsiness.
- Demonstrate Marked Changes in Gait.
- Show Poor Coordination in Group Games.

Secondary symptoms or related phenomena may include:

- Being the Last to Be Chosen on Teams (unless he has a *strong* prior history of athletic success or sustained friendships).
- Having Poor Navigational Skills.
- Having Poor Stamina on Walking Trips and Field Trips. May Lag Behind Others and May 'Sit Out' Activities.

Note:

- ➢ Some difficulties stem from increased dysfunction in vestibular integration (having to do with balance), fine motor ability, and language processing.
- ➢ Over time, lack of exercise may, in turn, affect former abilities to attend, learn, and respond to stress.[19]

11. Fine Motor Skills

❖ In a study of youth with PANDAS, a marked impairment in fine motor speed was associated with Group A beta-hemolytic Streptococcus titer elevations.[20]

Indications of difficulties in this area may include the following:

- Handwriting Regresses to Look Like That of One Much Younger.
- Work Becomes Difficult for Others to Read.
- Written Work Takes Much Longer to Complete than with Peers.
- Math Calculation Work is Poorly Organized (i.e., adding long sums, long division, factoring, writing long formulas, transferring).
- Drawings of People Become Typical of a Student who is Years Younger.
- The Ability to Copy Material Is Reduced from blackboard or from other work.
- Written Products are Poorly Organized (i.e. margins and spacing of words and lettering are less uniform and clear.)
- Art Work is at a Regressed Level and Quality, including drawings, crafts, and sewing, etc.
- The Ability to Move or to Manipulate Objects[21] for the Purpose of Organizing or Tidying Up is Regressed (such as wrapping a garden hose around a reel in the school garden, buttoning, repairing. or hanging up clothes, or folding flags, blankets, or other materials.
- Overall Academic Fluency is Decreased. He or she needs more time to do the same amount of reading, writing, and math tasks, etc., as peers.
- Is Observed to be a "*Messy Eater.*" Less fluent and coordinated in the use of napkins and eating utensils.
- The Ability to Use Manipulatives is Regressed, or Weakened in the use of their own drawings, symbols, etc. as learning tools.

Drawings That Demonstrate Loss of Fine Motor Skills During Acute Illness

Before Symptom Onset | **During Acute Episode**

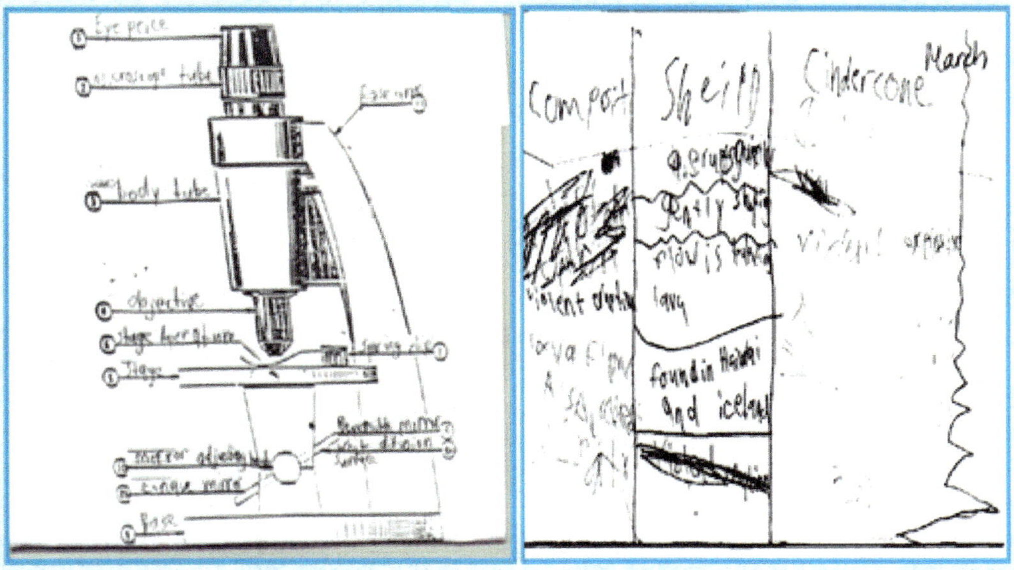

(Taken from Swedo SE, Leckman, and JF Rose NR (2012) From Research Subgroup to Clinical Syndrome Modifying the PANDAS Criteria to Describe PANS (Pediatric Acute-onset Neuropsychiatric Syndrome) Pediatrics and Therapeutics 2:113.)

12. Memory

- **Short term**, **long term**, and **working memory** may all be affected.
- **Working memory** is defined as the ability to hold information in one's immediate awareness while performing a mental operation on the information.[22]

Students with memory challenges may exhibit the following:

- Poor Rate of Task Completion.
- Incomplete or Missing Homework (where formerly was complete).
- Poor or Very Slow Math Calculation and Skills (weaker/slower memory for formulas, steps, ways of solving problems.
- Seemingly Weaker Abstract Reasoning. (Does not seem as quick to 'make connections' as previously.
- Worsened Time Management Skills.
- Poor Ability to Recall Details of Long Read ng Passages.
- During 'Waxing' Phases May Experience Sensory Overload, which can both color and limit what he remembers during that time.
- Weakened or Slower Ability to Make Decisions. Poor ability to recall *details,* and then to effectively synthesize and act on that information, especially when *sustained attention and processing speed* are both required.

- Poor Ability to Remember Multi-Step Directions.
- Limitations In Communicating What Is Causing Oneself Discomfort or Stress. (Students with PANS, especially the younger students, may be unable to articulate why they are uncomfortable. This may stem from poor articulation and social language skills. At times, it may occur because they are still in a 'reactive' mode to whatever is bothering them. Moreover, such limitations may also stem from a poor memory retrieval of how they felt *before* the onset of PANS symptoms. As a result, they may not be able to fully assimilate and compare those experiences to what they are feeling *now*.)

Note:

> Memory loss may also be affected by lack of sleep and stress. (Poor quality and quantity of sleep can especially affect long term memory.)
> General fatigue, ill health, and interrupted sleep patterns can affect attention and memory. [23]

..So, How Would One Use *Working Memory*?

A good example of the use of working memory is the ability to solve a long division problem without the use of pen and paper. For most people, as the *amount* to be divided and the *divisor* become larger (say, 498/29) it will become increasingly difficult to both *remember* quotients (and remainders) derived for previous columns, *and* engage in the mental process of dividing what's in the *next column*.

There are a variety of tests that are used to measure working memory. One type of assessment requires that the listener 'reorder' a list of items that he or she has just heard. (Reordering might involve now going from smallest to largest, numerically, etc.). In this case, one needs to both *remember* the items on the list **and** *mentally manipulate* that information at the same time, all without the 'memory-assist' of pen and paper.

In this last type of testing (that primarily requires *auditory* working memory for short bursts of time) measurements of 'working memory' can be deceiving. In this case, the student with PANS *may* be able to summon the energy, attention, and memory skills to do well, especially if no fine motor skills or much visual processing are needed. However, going back to what we know about PANS and the onset of visual processing difficulties, working memory can predictably be thwarted if tasks also involve eye/ hand coordination, or the processing of multiple images (especially if they are presented in quick succession). With this in mind, consider tests for working memory that require visual processing and auditory processing given in *isolation of one another*, *simultaneously*, and then, *with fine motor demands* added (like writing or peg work).

13. Speech and Language Challenges

Indications of difficulties in this area can include:

- Regression in Social Language similar to that of a younger person, including unexpected "baby talk."
- Changes in Conservational Turn-Taking; Increasing is Missing 'Social Cues,' etc.
- Oral Motor Changes (i.e., hyper-salivating, changes in the way the mouth moves, messy eating).
- Unexpected Voice Changes in tone pitch or volume, or weakened articulation of words, or sounds.
- Slower Speech Rate/Fluency.
- Weakened Sense of Humor. Weaker ability to formulate/and or process verbal jokes than before.
- Inability to Articulate What is Causing Discomfort or Stress.

- Insertion of Unexpected Sounds, Breaks or Movements in Spoken Language (including vocal or physical tics).
- Repetitive "copycat" exclamations, as seen in a form of OCD called *echolalia*, or random, frequent interruptive utterances.

Secondary symptoms or related phenomena may include:

- Increased Fear or Total Avoidance of Public Speaking.

Note:

- The stakes get higher with age. Peers are continuing to move forward in all areas of language development, including the understanding of language nuances, metaphors, humor, and sarcasm, etc.
- At the same time, many of these students will be able to *maintain*[24] a good vocabulary (even if they do not always fully articulate, or use that vocabulary in ways that are expected in conversations).

14. Social Skills and Interactions

Indications of changes in this area can include:

- Strained Relationships with friends and acquaintances.
- Verbal or Physical Attacks by others, resulting from reduced capacity to 'read' and to respond to body language or language nuances.
- Reduction in Social Interactions.
- Peers Avoid Being Near the Student and consistently sit in other areas.
- Taunting, Bullying, Stigmatizing, and Social Isolation by others, as a result of PANS- associated behaviors (such as verbal tics or compulsive spitting, etc.). Unfortunately, this may include actions or words of peers, but also those of teachers and others in authority.[25]
- Student Begins to Seek Out Relationships Outside of 'Peer Group.' These may include acquaintances with older or younger aged individuals, children from other countries, or peers otherwise outside of the 'mainstream' social group. Often, such individuals might be seen as more accepting, offering the 'benefit of the doubt' (or not noticing altogether) certain behaviors that same-aged peers might find fault in.
- Student Demonstrates Difficulty when Participating in 'Cooperative Learning Activities,' where teams of students are working together. This student may be slow to respond to or keep up with others, or he may not be able to do 'his part' on the team. The student may not know what his part in the group-driven product is, or should be; yet he may have great difficulty asking for clarification. He may encounter criticism by team members who fear they will have to cover for him, or in effect, do his work for him.[26]
- Student Shows Aggression if there is a need to "save face" as social awareness heightens.
- Student Exhibits Loss of Verbal Skills, Hyperactivity, and Explosive Behavior- Some students can become assaultive, impatient, and demanding, all in an effort to calm their anxiety and "get what they need" to fulfill a compulsion or obsession.

Note:

- May continue to interact appropriately (for short amounts of time) with trusted adults (teachers, therapists, medical providers, and others), *especially in waning periods of the disease.*
- Same aged peers may be the first to notice irregularities in PANS' sufferers.[27]

15. <u>Sensory Defensiveness (and Under Sensitivity)</u>

- Sensory Defensiveness includes aspects of Tactile, Auditory, Visual, Olfactory, and other sensory feedback systems.
- Some may experience *under sensitivity*, which can result in 'cravings' for increased feedback from those sensory systems.

Students with challenges in this area may:

- <u>Use Protective Mechanisms and Responses</u> (such as placing hands over ears) to shield oneself from loud or uncomfortable noises.
- <u>Refuse to Be around Different People or Objects</u> that make certain sounds, tones, pitches, etc.
- <u>Indicate Discomfort with Changes in Lighting</u>, bright lights, or florescent lights.
- <u>Show Irritability (or Other Notable Reactivity) in Response to Sudden Changes in Lighting.</u>
- <u>Show Reactivity to Certain Odors.</u>
- <u>Indicate Reactivity and Discomfort with Certain Textures and Articles of Clothing.</u> May be wearing similar types of clothing over long periods, perhaps due to restricted clothing requisites based on poor or unusual tactile response to items. Reports of hearing that for this student, all clothing, including socks and underwear, have to feel "just right."
- <u>Demonstrate Difficulty Navigating Position in Space</u> due to poor sensory integration of vision and tactile perception.
- <u>Show Atypical Reactivity to Drafts</u> (wanting less or wanting more).
- <u>Have Difficulty with Movement</u> (as in riding in vehicles, including school busses). Reports of students feeling "trapped" in vehicles.[28]
- <u>Be Messy Eaters.</u> Moreover, may not be aware of food particles on face and clothes.
- <u>Demonstrate an Inability to Integrate Sensory Information from Different Sources *Simultaneously*</u> (such as seeing, hearing, and moving) in an efficient manner.
- <u>May Look Overwhelmed on Bus Rides.</u> May be sitting entirely by himself on field trips.
- <u>Demonstrate Taste and Olfactory Reactiveness</u> surrounding discomfort and irritation with certain odors and tastes.
- <u>Suck Constantly on Shirts and/or Fingers</u> (especially noted in younger children. This is assumed to be regressive behavior).
- <u>Show Unusual Reactivity</u> to certain chemicals, cleaning solvents, electromagnetic sensitivity, or other suspected or unknown triggers.
- <u>Show Indications of Cravings</u> may include the need for strong or continued tastes (like lime water or peppermint), odors, tactile feedback (such as rabbit's foot or set of keys), and rocking.
- <u>Poke, Touch, or Prod</u> items or people in a manner that is atypical for age or peers.
- <u>Jump up and down</u> as if to "shake off" agitation.

Note:

- Severe sensory defensiveness may look indistinguishable from anxiety, panic attacks, or OCD behaviors.

16. Vestibular Dysfunction

- Vestibular *dysfunction* concerns the inefficient processing of information having to do with movement, space, and gravity.
- Vestibular *function* is generally associated with the sense of balance.[29]
- Efficient vestibular function allows the eyes to focus when the head is moving. (A figure skater doing spins would very likely have outstanding vestibular function.)
- Inefficient processing of movement, space, and gravity can result in Vestibular *hyper* (or over) sensitivity, or *hypo* (or under) sensitivity.

***Hyper**sensitivity* to vestibular movement in the learning setting may result in the following:

- Negative Reactions to Movement on swings, merry-go-rounds, or other rides (associated with vestibular hypersensitivity and gravitational insecurity).
- A Formerly Active Student now 'Sitting on the Side,' rather than physically engaging in recreational sports activities.
- The Student Becomes Notably Anxious and Uncomfortable Around Climbing and Playground Equipment.
- The Youth Becomes Nauseous, Irritable, or Appears 'Overwhelmed' in Cars.

***Hypo**sensitivity* to vestibular movement in the learning setting may result in an *increased* tolerance for movement, and result in the following.

- A Student Appears to Seek out Activities that Provide Vestibular Sensations, such as going too fast or dangerously on playground equipment.
- May Appear Hyperactive, or Takes on 'High Risk' Activity compared to same aged peers.

17. Propioceptive Dysfunction

- When defined, propioceptive *dysfunction* is usually associated with tactile and/or vestibular difficulties).
- Pertains to difficulties in interpreting body position and movement sensations.
- When an individual is stopped by the police to determine if they are intoxicated, he may be given a *Field Sobriety test* (which basically measures proprioception.)

Students who have difficulty in this area may:

- Display Poor Body Awareness.
- Display Motor Control Difficulties and Poor Motor Planning.
- Use Poor Manipulation of Objects (such as 'learning objects' or manipulatives that are used as tools to learn concepts (Cuisenaire rods for math, charts for science experiments, etc.)
- Be Increasingly 'Clumsy.'
- Appear to be a Messy Eater.

- Demonstrate Poor Grooming Skills.
- Demonstrate Sensory Seeking Behaviors such as jumping up and down (as if to "shake off" agitation), bumping into other children, and prodding, touching, and poking, etc.

Happy Times in the Family Car

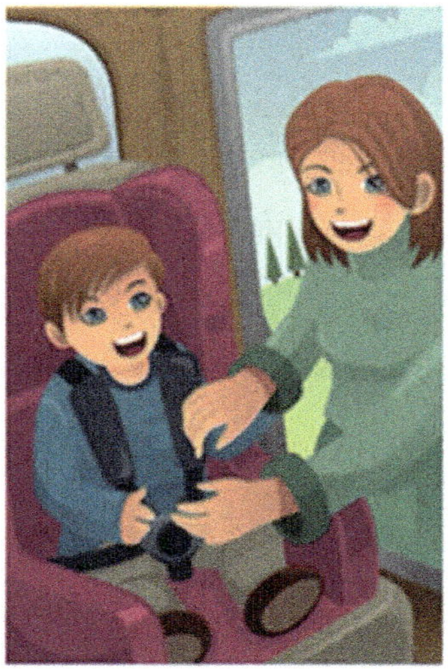

(...Not!)

A Potentially Perfect Storm of Tactile, Propiocentric, Vestibular, Auditory, Visual, and Other Sensory Dysfunction, Accentuated by the Probable Overlay of Obsessions, Compulsions, Attentional Limitations, 'Sickness Behavior,' and Other Factors...

J. Candelaria Greene (2014)
(Photo credit illustrator: artisticco, 2015, with thanks to Reese Bretow

18. Enuresis (Surrounding the Need to Urinate Frequently)

Indications that students may have difficulties in this area include the following:

- They Take Frequent Trips to the Bathroom (which can be prompted by physical or psychological concerns).
- Others Note Wetness on Pants.
- There is Reluctance and Concern (by Parents) for their Children to Attend Activities/Fieldtrips that are not near a bathroom. (Will there be a toilet on the field trip bus or sufficient bathroom stops on the way? Will the event have accessible toilets for students to use? Who will accompany the student to the bathroom, when necessary?)
- There is an Increase in the Use of Liners, especially among younger students.
- Students Move in Such a Way that Indicates the Need to Go to the Bathroom.
- Disposable Diapers or Heavy Liners Are Needed to Attend Overnight Trips.
- There is a Distinct Odor of Urine (or Feces) When in Close Proximity.
- There are Reports of Excessive Bed Wetting In Older Children (over the age of ten especially).

19. Grades and Performance

Changes can include the following:

- Report Cards Reveal a Jagged Profile. High and low grades and scores in the same subject throughout the semesters and years.
- Winter Quarter Report Card Scores May be Weaker/Lower (secondary to increased exposure to infection).
- Math Scores May be Lower/Higher (correlating with waxing and waning of symptoms).
- There may be Significant Waxing and Waning Patterns in Multi-Year Review of Bench Mark Scores (i.e., California STAR Testing), especially if tests were timed.

Note:

> Sometimes high scores and grades on such records may be deceptive. Whereas one would expect to see lower grades during times of waxing PANS symptoms, they may appear to stay the same. However, this may be only due to the assistance of loved ones, tutors, or school staff, etc, who are stepping in and providing intense levels of support. Also, consider other factors, such as changes facilitated by an intervening IHP, 504, or IEP that were put into place, or changes in placement from advanced level (AP) classes to basic classes that are less difficult, etc.

A Closer Look at The Complex Skills of Language and Executive Functioning Or: Task *Efficiency May be only as Good as Its Weakest Requisite Skills will Allow*

As we have just seen, PANS affects a number of human functions that are required to learn and to participate in the educational setting. In fact, the degree to which this interplay of different physical and mental skills can efficiently work together will, in large part, determine one's ability to learn, demonstrate, and maintain academic skills.

These include some of the more obvious behaviors, such as weakened abilities to execute gross motor movements (like skipping) and fine motor movements (such as writing with a pencil). It may include subtle or profound differences in speech articulation, or avoidance of certain sounds or lights, or a noticeable aversion to moving too fast on swings or slides.

However, there are many functions during the school day that require a student to employ a broad number of skills *simultaneously.* This, of course, means that, to the extent that *one* or more parts of this multifaceted mechanism is not working well, the more likely the completion of the whole task will be compromised, or at least, slowed down.

The Complex Feat of Language

Let's look first at the example of language skills. **Language** is generally thought of in terms of ***expressive*** **language** (that includes vocabulary, how one articulates words, etc.), and ***receptive*** **language**, that generally refers to how well the person understands what others have said. However, human language cannot be so neatly summed up as 'output' and 'input.'

If one were to do a 'discourse analysis' of a conversation between a 'neurotypical student' and a student suffering from PANS, for example, one might notice differences in such **quantitative** features as length, speed, and number of words uttered by each student. One would likely note **qualitative** differences too. For example, the listener might perceive differences in enthusiasm, energy levels, or even indications of sarcasm (indicated by changes in pitch, tone, and rhythm). In addition, one might note affirmative acknowledgements as well (such as laughter, or expressions, such as, *"Oh Yeah!"* or *"Right!"*). One could also take note of the choice of subject matter, and the ability to link or 'mirror' what the previous speaker said, to what the next speaker said.

Then, if one were to view a videotape of the interaction, one could glean even more about the student's language skills. One might notice, for example, that this student is not making eye contact with his peer. He might be frowning, or looking away, or shuffling his feet. Unlike most speakers in conversation, this student may not be mirroring the other student's movements (like smiling or nodding) or giving other visual indications that he is staying engaged.

Lastly, the observer might notice changes in movement and facial expressions that, along with a few words (by either student) would signal an abrupt end to the conversation.

Underlying reasons for such differences and changes in social language could result from a number of PANS symptoms. These could include such factors as fatigue, changes in articulation, or even other factors (such as an unspoken need to go to the bathroom). Weakened visual processing skills can also play a role in such conversational changes. Whereas such students might still excel in activities where they can look at stationary images (such as chess boards, where pieces stay put for short periods of time), they may miss sequences of visual information that are presented quickly.[30] While this could include the processing of movies, or the recall of specific buildings when traveling by in a car, it could also include the interpretation of rapid visual sequences presented in body language. As a result, these students might not be reading body language, or processing other visual signals as quickly and efficiently as they used to.[31] Moreover, '**inner speech**,' described as a form of *internalized, self-directed dialogue*,[32] can undergo a metamorphosis in these students, whereby an onslaught of new feelings and feedback from others (from conversations such as these) combine to reshape their world. Predictably then, for many of these students, as the number of verbal exchanges accumulates in a given day, so do their requisite demands for acceptable articulation, fluency, memory, physical and verbal 'mirroring,' word retrieval, attention, visual processing, and self-censure. With each successive encounter, then, he or she becomes at higher risk of faltering in some aspect of the exchange- resulting in errors, misunderstandings, and worse, humiliation. It is no wonder then, for many students who are in the depths of this illness, that verbal exchanges can become increasingly limited.

...And the Equally Complex Feat of Executive Function

Our second example surrounds the complex demands required for **Executive Function.** Executive Function is typically associated with those skills necessary to plan, organize, and successfully execute an activity under a given timeline. It is also associated with the regulation of attention, emotion, and social functioning.[33]

Susanne Phillips Keeley[34] characterizes executive function disorders as including the following:

- difficulty with planning and organization
- trouble identifying what needs to be done
- problems determining the sequence of accomplishment
- difficulty carrying out the steps in an orderly way
- difficulty beginning tasks
- problems maintaining attention
- trouble evaluating how they are doing on a task
- difficulty taking feedback or suggestions

Markers of good executive functioning include the ability to shift mental sets and tasks efficiently, and the ability to inhibit ones verbal and behavioral responses as needed (in social and other situations).[35]

Greater facility in executive functioning is largely developmental in nature, in that as the brain develops, the expanding prefrontal area of the brain allows for greater reasoning ability, prediction, abstraction, sustained attention, self-regulation, and working memory. These skills and more, combined with a solid knowledge base gleaned from real-world experience, make for seamless executive function.

How would executive function affect one's ability to navigate one's life on a day to day basis? In light of the indispensable role that executive function plays in the management[36] of PANS, its description and effects bear a closer look. Towards this end, the following two portraits are presented. In one, this skill set allows for spectacular success. In the other, it offers independence, survival, and hope.

Chronicles of Very Good Executive Functioning

Part 1: Margaret Hosts a Gathering... and a Wedding

One stellar example of an *Executive-Function Extraordinaire* is Margaret. Years ago, this marvelous woman spearheaded the founding of a small 'Consult' group for Bay Area learning specialists. Her devoted efforts included the offering up of her posh San Francisco home in which to meet. On the second Saturday of each month, professional updates, research findings, and suggested strategies for case studies would be reviewed. This would then be followed by an hour of delightful conversation and light (but scrumptious) refreshment.

On this one spring morning, as the group chatted away between bites of *petit fours* and sips of *Peets,* a question emerged from one of the attendees. Wasn't her daughter getting married sometime soon? And how *were* the preparations going on that front?

Taking a sip of her tea before gracefully placing the cup back on its porcelain saucer, this perfectly *ensembled* matriarch began. Her brief, but nevertheless warm and engaging response recounted *just enough* for any listener to 'fill in the blanks.' Clearly, this had been a strong mother-daughter collaboration, where over the span of many months, an abundance of creativity, planning, problem solving, and knowledge of resources, all combined to ensure that both the wedding and reception were going to be lovely, memorable, and grand affairs.

Her enthralled listeners recognized at once that the Cathedral and world-famous hotel (where the reception would be held) required a reservation to be placed *at least* a year in advance. The renowned caterer and musicians, *ditto*. And then, wasn't the groom's family from Sweden? *No problem.* With Margaret at the helm, any and all aspects of religious and cultural views would be researched, thoughtfully considered, and appropriately addressed. To be sure, *not 'just addressed;'* the resulting nuptials would be a glittering melding of traditions, customs, and beliefs precious to *both* families. It would undoubtedly be Margaret too, with her knowledge of various protocols,[37] guest personalities, and verbal finesse and discretion, who would masterfully designate the seating arrangements of the (over) two hundred guests. Unintentional offense (or the appearance of exclusion) to anyone on this special occasion would simply not happen.

Side discussions of '*The Wedding*' now rippled through the room. Several attendees were heard to marvel on her insertion of a distinct *Impressionist* theme. (The newlyweds would be honeymooning in Paris, with a side trip planned for Giverny[38]). The rest of us sat back in our surprisingly comfortable *Mission-style* cushioned seats, reflecting on this fairy tale event to come. "Wow..." was the sole expression that echoed among the ranks.

The final stroke of noon chimed decisively from the antique Grandfather clock in the hall, signaling the end to another splendid (and actually productive) gathering. As we wended our way out through her camellia garden to our waiting cars, we continued to listen attentively, as the 'new comer' to the group asked our hostess what no one else had thought to ask. It was then that we collectively froze to a stunned silence as Margaret responded- *decidedly rather calmly to our minds*- "Oh, a little later this afternoon."

And there it is. *How*, one might ask, could *any* woman so confidently secure the completion of an infinite number of tasks[39] under such unforgiving time lines, to the point that she could even *think* about hosting a meeting of associates in the morning, and a *wedding*, (much less, her *daughter's*) in the afternoon?

Three words: *Outstanding Executive Function.*

Chronicles of Very Good Executive Functioning

Part 2: Sheldon, Melvin, and Adrian (Or, What do These Guys Have that Our Kids Don't?)

Now, let us shift the lens away from a very real, albeit rare, *'Executive Function Extraordinaire,'* to the examples of three men- all fictitious, but in their way, exemplary in how each draws on the gifts of executive function to effectively manage his often difficult internal and external environments.

Messrs. *Sheldon Cooper,*[40] *Adrian Monk,*[41] and *Melvin Udall* [42] are men whose lives are all, in some way, constricted by fears, compulsions, and overwhelm of various sorts. All three, for example, suffer from phobias surrounding contamination and/or germs. Melvin Udall, for instance, the gifted writer depicted in the movie *"As Good As It Gets,"* is seen to carry his own disposable utensils- in the possible event that he may need to eat out. We also observe how our brilliant Detective Monk, from the television comedy of the same name, quickly becomes disturbed if personal items have been moved- even *slightly* askew. Of note too, all three gentlemen have been known to complete rituals where numbers, names, or actions are repeated.

It's plausible that our illustrious Dr. Sheldon Cooper, the lead character of the popular television show *"The Big Bang Theory"* may also show indications of sensory integration overwhelm/dysfunction too. He becomes easily distressed, for example, as the raised tones and volumes of arguing come within hearing range. The act of hugging another (undertaken only under the most extreme of circumstances) is transacted as stiffly as possible, and then, with only the most deliberate and measured efforts. It is further fair to say that, although a long time resident of highway-ladened California, Sheldon (like the good Detective Monk) neither wishes, nor is likely well suited, to drive a car. We discover that a prior attempt at learning to drive- which of course requires the efficient and simultaneous processing of multiple sensory data at once- has resulted in several crashes and the assumed demise of innocent bystanders. (Fortunately for the citizens of this fictionalized town of Pasadena, however, such crashes actually take place on his friend Howard's computerized driving-simulation-program, and not a real car.)

In these stories then, each man's days are constricted by surges of various internal and external mandates and limitations. However, a closer look at the lives of Sheldon, Adrian, and Melvin reveals some rather noted accomplishments nonetheless. We discover that all three not only attended secondary school, but likely completed college as well. They have been actively engaged in, and successful in, their chosen professions, and for many years. They all live independently from their parents, are responsible for their own finances, and maintain very good housekeeping skills (as evidenced by scenes of tidy and organized dwellings). Last, but not least, our protagonists all appear to be well groomed and healthy. Clearly they are eating enough and of the right foods, and arrange to have at least adequate amounts of health care.

How are these men able to navigate their lives, in ways that allow them to be at least *functional* (if not always at peace with the world)? To answer this question, let's go back to their respective story lines and pluck out a few clues. For one thing, they are all adults, both *legally*, and *physically*. In addition to having the requisite intellectual abilities and knowledge base to do so, both Adrian and Melvin also have the financial resources to *live alone.* [43] Living alone allows each to know (with a high level of confidence), that for one thing, no uninvited entity will be touching, 'contaminating,' or moving their things without their knowledge or permission. Although it is true that Sheldon does share an apartment (a two bedroom), with "Leonard," he also can take comfort in the knowledge that at any time, he can draw upon his 75 item (plus)[44] "roommate agreement,"[45] should any deviation from the 'expected and planned' transgress. This document, of course, details the scheduled times for each party to use the bathroom each morning, contingencies for changing prior agreements, (i.e., the assigned order of restaurants on their strictly designated weeknights,[46]) and compacts for Leonard to drive him (Sheldon) to work.

As far as addressing any contamination concerns, specifically, we can count on Adrian and Melvin to do the necessary task analysis to plan for such eventualities, and thus, come to restaurants fully prepared. Whereas Melvin brings disposable utensils along, Adrian brings a hired assistant (who will also have all the necessary decontamination supplies at the ready).

We see then, that each of our heroes is equipped with the requisite skills to consider, predict, plan, and prepare for situations that even *might* cause him *future* distress. With the gifts of time, maturity, and experience, each one has also been able to learn, synthesize, and incorporate new information too, regarding the potential use and effectiveness of any 'self-protective measures.' These exquisite skill sets, the hallmark of good executive functioning, afford these men, at the very least, the promise of *functional lives*, if not the 'ideal lives' their viewers hope for them.

Moreover, Sheldon's, Melvin's, and Adrian's very good executive function, each made possible by a fully developed prefrontal lobe, allows these men to have a sense of *control* and *agency*, as they strive to negotiate their day to day lives. Again, not to be underestimated are their intellectual and financial capabilities, and generally good physical health overall, that will certainly help facilitate their journeys through life. That said, it will be their finely honed *executive function* that will be the ultimate determinant, in not only their ability to maintain stewardship of their own lives, but in the possible recognition, remediation, and eventual *diminishment* of their respective psychological burdens too.[47]

And Now, Back to the Real World...

In strong contrast to the real-life *Margaret* and the make-believe creatures of *Sheldon et al,* PANS-stricken youth are impacted by debilitations that at once make them needy for effective coping mechanisms, while at the same time, less able in fact, to construct or to draw from such mechanisms. *Executive Functioning,* a crucial piece in the development and execution of effective coping skills, is both underdeveloped *and* thwarted in these students. This is a result of their, not only, still-developing and immature brain (along with compromised memory and inner language), but from a relative lack of real world knowledge and experience (along with other obvious deficiencies, such as an obvious lack of financial and other resources, etc.) Combined with the manifestations of the sickness behavior itself,[48] it is no wonder that these youths are ill prepared to take on the overall management of their various impairments, much less a sudden onset of disturbing feelings and unexpected behaviors, too.

In fact, a major theme that quickly emerges in conversation with parents and family members of students with PANS surrounds the loss of executive functioning.[49] This loss results in the parent taking on a tremendous logistical load in order for the child to complete many basic functions and tasks of daily living. Without their prior abilities to efficiently think, plan, coordinate, and organize their world and their lives, these children succumb to- for all intents and purposes- developmental regression.[50]

Such developmental and functional immaturity even extends to how the student is able to form a **perspective**, or point of view, with regard to his circumstances, ideas, etc. What are the building blocks of a perspective that is rational, thoughtful, and purposeful? Key elements include executive function, language, and memory, that all must effectively combine to allow for perspective's requisite skills of observation, reflection, and synthesis to take place.

Psychiatrist Dr. Daniel Siegel describes the term *Mindfulness* as an "integrated state of mental processing, that involves a wide range of attentional, emotion regulating, conceptual and observational processes that are harnessed in a flexible and adaptive manner."[51] As these young people strive to make sense of, and navigate their way through this often life-changing condition, a *mindful perspective* becomes essential and pivotal, sometimes to their very survival.

...And Last, but Not Least, the (Not Always Observable) Changes *Outside* of the School Setting

PANS-stricken families, not unlike their affected children, will be impacted in very differently ways. As with other families of loved ones with critical needs, family members strive to do what is possible to help their students prepare to be ready and alert for the school day. In the case of a child with PANS, however, this often entails huge levels of support,[52] which can put tremendous demands on all family members. This is especially true for the primary care provider, who must suddenly, and incessantly, orchestrate and deliver large amounts of medical care, educational support, and other interventions as needed.[53] As a result, this caregiver's stress-burden can be very heavy. For the entire family, however, such stressors can also prove overwhelming, even for the healthiest of families.

The effectiveness of such management can be thwarted by a number of factors. Although rarely acknowledged, it can even be thwarted by beliefs surrounding this primary caretaker's perceived (and actual) degree of power and agency within the family and society. Like anyone else, this twin pairing of unspoken beliefs and assumptions will be largely shaped by upbringing, age, education, experience, and specific cultural and social expectations. Along with that parent's own unique inner sense of resolve and resilience, such perceptions combine to determine how she or he will go about communicating with others, including those in positions of 'authority.'[54] Moreover, when necessary, these exchanges will also include the generally unpleasant tasks of negotiating, advocating, questioning, and confronting others on behalf of their ill child.

There are a host of other factors too that pose constraints on the family's ability to help their child through this crisis. Nonetheless, as reflected in the interdependent triad of the school, home, and student, it will fall to the collective buttressing of the family, with the primary care taker at its helm, that will ultimately determine the nature of this child's academic fate.[55]

Especially during times of illness and symptom exacerbation then, and whether or not it is observed by the school staff, it should be considered a given that in these families, loved ones are providing their child with very high levels of support to bolster whatever remaining function their child still has. As a result, the parents themselves are at an equally high risk of physical and emotional exhaustion.

With this in mind, there are a number of variables that can affect a family member's resilience and well-being, as their loved one's illness is addressed. Examples[56] include the following:

- The Length and Extent of the Illness.
- The Primary Care Giver's Understanding of the PANS mechanism (in terms of how it affects the child- especially regarding negative or unexpected behaviors).
- The ***Non-Primary Care Giver's*** Understanding of the PANS Mechanism. (In many families this is usually the other spouse or partner, but in some instances may include siblings and grandparents, etc.).
- The ***Non-Primary*** Care Giver's Trust, Support, and Communication with the primary care provider regarding the management and treatment of PANS, and its related symptoms. (As respondents indicated, despite the multifaceted and time-consuming nature of this care and health management, most of the primary care giver's day-to-day efforts can go largely unnoticed or unacknowledged by others, including other family members, who may not be at home when such support occurs).[57] In these instances it falls to other family members, but especially the non-primary care provider- to trust that the primary care provider is acting knowledgably and competently on the child's behalf, and that also she/he is doing the best s/he can under the circumstances.
- The Demands of Parental Careers, especially that of the primary care provider.
- The Ability to Negotiate Effectively and Candidly among all family members.
- The Accessibility, Trust, and Support of Extended Family Members.
- The Degree of Accordance among Treating Providers.
- The Availability of Financial and Other Resources for Securing the Following:
  - Medical insurance.
  - Appropriate medical and psychological care by knowledgeable providers.
  - Respite care for their child with PANS, and respite care for siblings.
  - Indirect support of the child, primary care provider, and family, including such time saving and supportive assistance as childcare and housecleaning.
  - Opportunities for the primary care giver to take care of her/himself, such as meeting with friends, or engaging in opportunities that bring contentment.
  - Opportunities for the parents to spend time and do activities with non-PANS children and other family members.
  - Opportunities for the student to remain in clubs, organizations, sports, and other activities (providing continued involvement of the student, and providing needed respite for the parent, even in cases where they may also be in attendance).

- The Ages and Needs of other Family Members.
- The Ways in Which the PANS Illness is Discussed, Explained to, Perceived, and Interpreted by Siblings. (Do siblings feel that they may become sick or change too? Do they feel responsible for 'holding the family together' during this time of crisis?)
- Support from Other Parents and Groups Associated with PANS.
- The Temperaments and Resilience of other Family Members.
- The Time, Expertise, Ability, and Sense of Agency/Power on the Primary Care-Giver's Part (usually the mother) to orchestrate help for her child and for other family members. Regarding agency, for example, does she feel empowered to speak to, negotiate with, and if necessary, confront and disagree with providers regarding the needs, treatment, and diagnosis of her child?
- The Degree of Writing, Reading, and Speaking Skills that, when necessary, include enough of the lexicon (such as terminology/ phrases etc.) of the medical or educational well enough to convey a sense of understanding and command of her child's needs.
- The Support Coming from other Sources that lead to a sense of well-being for that individual (such as meditation, social networks and spiritual connection).

Given the above variables, what might school staffs notice, in terms of changes in appearance and dynamics with parents and family members? The following lists some of the more common observations.

- Increased Phone Calls From Parents Voicing Concerns.
- Family Relations May Appear Strained.
- Parent May Begin to Bring Student to School where once the student walked, took the bus, or carpooled.
- Obvious Increase in Parental Assistance in Child's Homework.
- Substantial Increase in Parent to School Communication regarding homework, tests, student interactions, etc.
- The Focal Point of Conversations with School Staff Center on This Child, and not the Siblings. (Student becomes center point of family life.)
- Parents or Other Family Members Demonstrate Possible Symptoms of Post-Traumatic Stress Disorder. These may include parental reports of:
  - Disinterest in Activities They Once Enjoyed.
  - Trouble Concentrating and Staying with a Conversation Activity.
  - Having Trouble Sleeping.
  - Appearing Easily Irritated, Angry, or Startled.
  - Reporting, or Appearing to be, Always on Guard for Danger.
  - Distancing Themselves From Friends or Others.
  - Going Out of His or Her Way to Avoid Activities and Events that May Bring about Overwhelm/Meltdowns for the Child (even as he or she appears to be improving and far less sensitive in these areas.)
  - Appearing to Be Less Positive and Expressive Than Before.
  - Feeling Hopeless about the Future.
  - Negative Feelings about Themselves and Others.[58]
- Parent Reports Marital Strife over questions of diagnosis, child discipline, and obtaining appropriate care for child, especially amidst dwindling finances.
- Parent Reports Reduction in Work Hours by One or Both Parents.

- Mother May Look Exhausted, Overwhelmed, or Easily Distracted; may appear to be thinking of something else.
- Siblings May Appear Overwhelmed or Less Talkative.
- Siblings May Appear to be Resentful of Student and/or May Distance Themselves from Issues and Discussion Surrounding this Student (It bears noting that many other siblings may not.)
- Siblings May Strain to Keep Away From Affected Student, or May be Spending More Time than Expected with him or her at Recess or other breaks. (Siblings may be at higher risk of unintentional verbal and physical abuse. At the same time, they may also be the sole confident/ source of support for this child.)
- Family Reports that Vacations, Extracurricular Activities, and any 'Long Term Planning' Are Now on 'Hold.'
- In Talking with Parents, Priorities Regarding Educational Goals Begin to Change. Education becomes a distant third to physical health, safety of child and family, and psychological well-being.
- A Surge in Medication, Therapies, etc., raises questions re: **Münchausen Syndrome by Proxy**.
- The Primary Care-Taker Reports that Relations with Support Systems are becoming strained (These include other family members, school community, friends and extended family members).[59]

As symptoms of the illness play out, an appropriate educational plan will be necessary to support the student too. How can families and providers begin to move forward towards the development of such a plan? Section III offers a glimpse of the academic 'big picture' for these students; one that extends beyond the immediate crisis of their illness and treatment. It lays down the necessary preplanning/groundwork down that will support educational planning and the implementation of services later on. It also cautions how PANS is strikingly different from other disabling conditions that school districts tend to be mostly familiar with.[60]

Notes

---

[1] The PANS Survey (in appendices) from pandasnetwork.org, can also act as a reference point to suggest ways in which PANS can disrupt daily activities. With thanks to Diana Pohlman for her excellent feedback on this section and for pandasnetwork.org for the inclusion of the survey.

[2] Candelaria Greene, JF (2015) Unpublished survey of family members, providers, and survivors of PANS regarding PANS and Education (2013-2015), collected as UC Berkeley Visiting Researcher Scholar, Berkeley, California.

[3] See Tona, J. & Posner, T. (2011) PANDAS/PITAND Recognizing and treating children with Pediatric Autoimmune Neuropsychiatric Disorders in OT. From: nysota information on PANDAS-PITAND and OT.

[4] Murphy, T. K., Patel, P. D., McGuire, J. F., Kennel, A., Mutch, P. J., Parker-Athill, E. C., Hanks, C. E., Lewin, A. B., Storch, E. A., Toufexi, M. D., Dadlani, G. H., & Rodriguez, C. A. (2015). Characterization of the Pediatric Acute-Onset Neuropsychiatric Syndrome Phenotype Journal of Child and Adolescent Psychopharmacology. February 2015, 25(1): 14-25. doi:10.1089/cap.2014.0062.

[5] ibid.

[6] Hergüner, S., Kilinçaslan, A., Görker, I., & Tüzün, U. (2007) Serotonin-selective reuptake inhibitor-induced enuresis in three pediatric cases. J Child Adolesc Psychopharmacol. Jun;17(3):367-9.

[7] Extra sensitivity to criticism can especially be linked to an increase in generalized anxiety (as noted by Psychologist Linda C. Avery PhD, personal communication: 12/15.

[8] American Psychiatric Association (2013). Diagnostic and Statistical Manual of Mental Disorders (Fifth ed.). Arlington, VA: American Psychiatric Publishing. p 235.

[9] ibid.

[10] ibid.

[11] 'Nesting nature' has to do with those activities that typically take place at home, including eating, grooming, dressing, and sleeping.

[12] Also, good coping suppression of OCD/tic symptomatology can result in an increase of tension and immediate release of emotional and physical expression upon returning to a safe environment, such as the home.

[13] Candelaria Greene, (2015).

[14] Also see Dan Siegel MD The Mindful Brain: Reflection and Attunement in the Cultivation of Well-Being (W.W. Norton 2007)

[15] See Lewin, A.B., Storch, E.A., Mutch, P.J., and Murphy, T.K. (2011) Neurocognitive functioning in youth with pediatric autoimmune neuropsychiatric disorders associated with streptococcus. J Neuropsychiatry Clin Neurosci. 2011 Fall; 23(4):391-8. doi: 10.1176/appi.neuropsych. 23.4.391.

[16] ibid.

[17] See also Section VI on accommodations as well.

[18] Dr. Mark Anderson, Clinical Optometrist, UC Berkeley School of Optometry (consult 1/19/2016).

[19] Continued opportunities for exercise become very important for PANS-stricken students, especially as we continue to learn more about how *prolonged stress levels* can affect gene expression. For example, in her research on RNA and 'alternative splicing,' Daniela Kaufer shows how, in the case of chronic exposure to increased levels of stress hormones (glucocorticoids), RNA's influence can result in the cell responding more rapidly than before. This in turn, can affect learning capacity and heighten fearfulness. However, exercise, along with yoga and meditation, have the potential to actually 'reset this molecular machinery' involved with stress response. (As noted in Lehrman, Sally (2008) *Nurture into Nature Meet Your New Brain*) Cal Alumni magazine Volume 119(2) March/April.)

[20] Lewin, A. B., Storch, E. A., et al, 2011, pp 391-8.

[21]Such as in the construction of a *California Mission* for a 4th grade History project to learn about California History, or the use of Cuisenaire rods used in Math to represent ones, tens, and 100's place, etc.

[22] Woodcock, R. W., McGrew, K. S., & Mather, N. (2001) Woodcock,-Johnson III. Itaska, IL: Riverside Publishing.

[23] Cytokines (involved in the inflammation process) and noted by Murphy (2015) is also associated with fatigue. This can also affect attention and memory.

[24](Or, remember and understand *the meaning of* a broad vocabulary.)

[25] As special education teachers *at all levels* related to me during this study, a big part of their work is to assure that their students are placed in classes with instructors whom they believe will, at the very least, be kind and respectful to students. Much thought and great efforts are made to avoid instructors whom they suspect will create educational trauma/damage for their students.

[26] Clearly, there are many roles and steps involved with such group work. Participation may be compromised by a host of factors associated with PANS, including working memory, auditory processing, etc.

[27] However, few will have the sensitivity, conviction, or perceived permission to speak up.

[28] Candelaria Greene, 2015.

[29] It is important to rule out inner ear difficulties, such as ear infections, which may temporarily produce similar effects.

[30] Thus indicating a need for accommodating the student with visual "anchors" when engaged in this type of learning activity.

[31] PANS exacerbations are often associated with weakened visual processing skills, as noted in Lewin et al, 2011.

[32] (Associated with Lev Vygotsky) to describe a stage in language acquisition and the process of thought. According to Vygotsky, speech begins as a social medium and becomes internalized as inner speech or verbalized thought. See a more complete discussion of the role of inner speech and language acquisition in Nelson K, & Bruner JS (2006). Narratives from the Crib. Cambridge, Mass: Harvard University Press.

[33] Siegel, D. J. (2008) The Mindful Brain: The Neurobiology of Well-Being. Boulder, Colorado: Sounds True Incorporated.

[34] Keeley, Susanne Phillips (2003) The Source for Executive Function Disorders. East Moline, IL: LinguiSystems.

[35] Blair, C., & Diamond, A. Biological processes in prevention and intervention: The promotion of self-regulation as a means of preventing school failure. Development and Psychopathology. 2008;20:899–911. [PMC free article] [PubMed]
[36] (And I would argue, *survivability* of this illness.)
[37] (Gleaned, we suspected, from all the volunteer work she did with fundraising efforts for the San Francisco Symphony and as a Maryknoll Lay Volunteer in previous summers.)
[38] Clearly associated with the garden and home of Impressionist artist Claude Monet.
[39] (This including the safeguarding of her own mental health).
[40] The character "Sheldon Cooper"(c) is featured on the American CBS Television Show 'The Big Bang Theory.'(2007-present)
[41] "Adrian Monk" (c) is the protagonist featured in the USA Network detective series entitled "Monk." (2002-2009)
[42] "Melvin Udall"(c) is one of the main characters in the movie "As Good as it Gets," (1997) produced by *Tri-Star Pictures* and *Gracie Films*.
[43] (For most of the story line)
[44] Not including its innumerable clauses, statutes, and amendments.
[45] Drawn up with utmost deliberation over many, many hours.
[46] One must not, for example, entertain the thought of going to a Thai restaurant on the weeknight reserved for pizza, etc.
[47] Not to be understated is the fact that, while the central dilemmas of these Hollywood characters get addressed in less than two hours, for many a PANS-stricken student, far more time and effort will be required.
[48] As noted in Murphy, 2015.
[49] Candelaria Greene, (2015).
[50] It is in this realm of Executive functioning, that school and teachers in particular can make a critical difference in how they accommodate for this student's needs.
[51] Siegel, D.G. Mindfulness training and neural integration: differentiation of distinct streams of awareness and the cultivation of well-being Soc Cogn Affect Neurosci 2007 2: 259-263. p. 261.
[52] As a parent of a child who recovered from PANS, health provider Ann Honigman, D.C., M.P.H. so perceptively observes, "Much of this would not be needed if the medical providers or health care system were to become knowledgeable about PANS. Upon diagnosis, there would be a roadmap of what to expect, support for the families and schools, and a heavy dose of hope that PANS is treatable. These recommendations would be viewed as temporary until which time, the student (would) be fully integrated back into their pre-PANS life."
[53] This is again where the school can lessen the tremendous load of the primary care taker and family through the use of 504's and IEPS's. Moreover, as one special education teacher stressed, "I always give families my cell number. Communication between the home and school is vital. After school homework help by a knowledgeable teacher is also helpful." (S.H. Consult, 11/1/15)
[54] For these reasons, it is helpful that the school, 504, or IEP team members "inventory" family dynamics, through interviews or informal communication.
[55] This signals the great need for any school team who is invested in the child's success to collaborate with the family in ways that will invariably lessen the stress on the primary giver as well.
[56] As reported by respondents (Candelaria Greene, 2015).
[57] Candelaria Greene, (2015).
[58] Of course, also review a fuller description and definition for PTSD under APA DSM IV and V. American Psychiatric Association. (2013). *Diagnostic and Statistical Manual of Mental Disorders* (5th Ed.). Washington, DC.
[59] Again, this underscores the need for respite care to be in place for this student.
[60] Of course, regardless of the diagnosis or disabling condition, as noted and seasoned special education teacher Stephanie Holeva emphasizes, "Ultimately... it is the individual needs of the student, *not the needs of a particular handicapping condition,* which should be addressed."

Section III

LAYING THE GROUNDWORK TO DETERMINE

EDUCATIONAL NEEDS AND OTHER SERVICES

Priorities Surrounding PANDAS/PANS in the Academic Setting

PANS manifests in intense symptoms that clearly threaten both the physical *and* psychological systems needed for learning. Therefore, when parents and providers begin to consider educational planning for their student with PANS, the following mandate and priorities should strongly be considered.

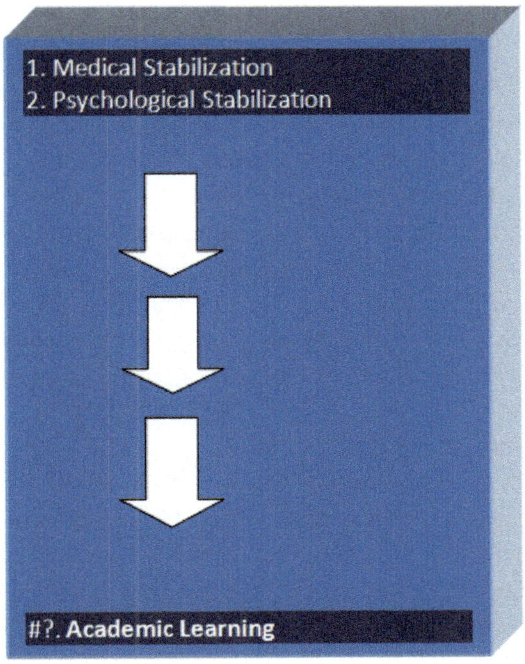

The graphic above represents two primary tenets regarding the student with PANS and academic planning.

First, the ability of this student to engage in an academic setting, or any other setting for that matter, will largely depend upon the degree to which medical and psychological symptoms have been addressed, or at the very least, *stabilized*. Moreover, the degree of the stabilization, and exacerbation of symptoms, will largely determine the *workable parameters* of the *what, where, when, and how* of this student's learning environment. For these reasons, the educational plan must hold tantamount any treatment and related supports for physical wellness first, with psychological wellness being an extremely close second. For it is only when these first two are bolstered and safeguarded, can the opportunity for academic learning really progress.

The second tenet surrounds the assumed mandate of *academic learning* for this youth. Up until now, the focal point of academics in their child's life has likely been seen as 'a given' in most families. As pointed out by parents and others interviewed,[1] prior to the onset of PANS, most of these students were not only able to engage in and negotiate a school setting, many of them clearly excelled in this environment. With the onset of such a health crisis as PANS, however, family expectations and priorities regarding academic learning (and its related markers of success), must suddenly descend to a lower place on the list of priorities. Moreover, in its worst manifestation, PANS can force families to dramatically alter their *expectations* of what their child is capable of, and rethink what milestones and accomplishments are now seen as feasible, or even important.

PANS-Stricken Families: Special Families within Special Families

Families of students with PANS have much in common with other families of students with special needs. For example, *unlike* the parents of "neurotypical/medically well" students, both sets of parents, typically the primary care providers will be spending far more time with, and for, their children- at doctors' appointments, therapy appointments, tutoring, transportation, assistance with skills of daily living and organization, etc... However, PANS' parents (along with the teachers who serve these children) struggle with some truly exceptional challenges on top of this.

First, the majority of students who are served for special learning needs tend to have conditions that are more pronounced in *one or two* domains. As an example, whereas students with ADHD are often found to have concommitant, or co-occurring conditions (such as ADHD, anxiety, or allergies, the *majority* do not have significant enough behavioral and medical issues that, on their own, would also qualify as an impairment to their participation in a learning environment. [2] [3] By definition though, the student with PANS not only suffers from a serious medical condition, but also from a debilitating set of behavioral/psychological/and developmental challenges- that are all happening *at the same time*.

Secondly, when considering the needs of most students with special needs, there is often an underlying assumption (based on the educator's experience) that such disabling conditions, like deafness, Trisomy 21 or Down Syndrome, and dyslexia, will generally be *stable over time* (in terms of how it affects the student's learning, behavior and participation in the classroom).[4] As a result, most providers and schools do not anticipate *substantial changes*- either positive or negative- in the short run (such as a few weeks or a few months). In contrast to these conditions, however, the calling card of PANS surrounds *sudden* and *jagged* debilitation across *multiple* domains. -At the same time though, and just as remarkably, the prognosis for this illness is nothing short of astoundingly positive. With appropriate treatment,[5] especially if provided early on in the disease process, a *complete recovery,* with accompanying reversal of cognitive, psychological, and physical debilitation, is entirely possible. Simply stated, in the world of Education and Special Education, it is rare to see such a phenomena of both *jagged and pervasive disability and profound recovery of abilities.*

Herein lies an unusual paradox for the school community then: *Despite the stunning incidence of one in two hundred children being affected,*[6] the condition is still very much an enigma to those providers and educators who are witnessing it for the first time. As such, it falls outside of the typical paradigm of treatment and remediation that most educational systems are familiar with, let alone are accustomed to working with. The nature of PANS can make planning and goal setting often challenging. This can be especially true among those school staffs that struggle to identify concrete absolutes, within such a universe of morphing and often eclipsing symptomatology such as PANS. Even in students who may have been affected for months or longer, and/or have less dramatic waxing and waning of symptoms, educational planning can be extremely challenging.

Consider then, how overwhelming it is for the parents of these children. They now, more than ever, depend upon communities of care (like the schools) to assist their child (and by extension their family) in their moment of need, only to discover that these communities may be fraught with misunderstandings and lack of knowledge regarding the nature of the disability itself. As a result, many PANS parents are thrust into the often awkward (and time-consuming) position of being the *de facto* 'specialist' in this regard, as they strive to help marshal in an appropriate plan of action. Adding to their challenge is that this is happening when they are already emboldened with the management of all the *other* aspects of this child's life, along with the coordination, care, and execution of other family responsibilities (such as employment and household care). As gleaned from parent and provider interviews,[7] no parent, no matter how loving, patient, resourceful, or even skilled professionally, can be prepared to anticipate, accommodate, and effectively address the myriad of needs that usually result from such demands.

Unique Educational Considerations for the Student with PANS

To be sure, addressing the educational needs of the student with PANS can be very overwhelming for families who are also juggling with a medical crisis at the same time. Other sections of this book will go into the process of obtaining accommodations, modifications, special education, and other supportive services. However, as the diagnostic and treatment processes surrounding PANS continue to unfold, parents and teachers should consider taking the following *initial steps* to support and safeguard their child's education.

Notifications of the School/Home

It is advisable that the parent, or guardian, notify the school regarding the presence of a medical (or any other type of condition) that could impair their child's participation in that school. This is important for a number of reasons. Regarding a medical condition or health concerns specifically, it is the practice of some school districts[8] to provide opportunities for modifications or home/hospital instruction--only *after* a medical absence (usually involving a minimum number of missed school days) has been established. In addition, as is clarified in the next chapter regarding related legislation, it is important to be mindful that even the *symptomatology* associated with PANS can warrant evaluations and services. At the very least, the parent might choose to telephone or email the teacher and/or principal/head mistress, and school office regarding what the family is seeing at home, and how it is presently being addressed.

Similarly, if teachers or staff members note student behaviors and inattention that are out of the ordinary for the student, it is very important to address these concerns with the parent, along with the school nurse or principal if possible. These observations can not only serve to validate some of the concerns over what the parent may be observing at home, but could also help initiate important referrals. Moreover, this exchange of information will help clarify *why* the behaviors are happening in the first place, so that other factors can be ruled out (such as 'indifference to learning,' or 'normal' student/peer upsets). Regardless of what the staff at school may be seeing, however, it bears noting that they're likely witnessing only a *milder version* of the type of symptoms that the family is dealing with at home.

Documentation Gathering and Other Important Information

Close collaboration with medical, mental health, and social service providers will also be important to consider as groundwork is being implemented. As much as possible, records and documents should be kept and put in designated areas. Sometimes the best one can do is to place them in separate folders/ binders/boxes for educational, medical, psychological, and other therapies, with the most recent document on the top. The most important consideration is to find what works in that parent's situation, so that documents can be retrieved when needed.

Considerations Regarding an Individualized Health Care Plan (IHCP)

In other chapters, we will review specific procedures for obtaining modifications, accommodations, and other interventions for this student. However, before steps are taken to implement those services, a request for an **Individualized Health Care Plan** should be considered. Depending upon where the student lives, this plan might also be referred to as an IHP (Individualized Health Plan), ICP (Individualized Care Plan) or something else.

Students with medical diagnoses such as Tourette Syndrome, OCD, or ADHD are often served under non-medical educational protocols such as **504**'s or **IEP**'s (which are formal educational plans that will be discussed further in Sections 4 and 5). For example, the parent might have documentation from the medical provider that their child has ADHD, and that it significantly impairs their ability to complete long tests in a room with multiple distractions. In this case, the student study team may initiate a 504 plan that would determine appropriate accommodations and/or special education. In addition, they would also very likely identify "ADHD" as the student's "**primary disabling condition**."[9]

However, the potentially broad reaching effects of a medical condition as severe as PANS demands that educational care and planning include some level of medical expertise at the *school* level, as well. For clearly, a diagnosis of PANS can be every bit as detrimental to educational achievement as other such potentially disabling conditions as diabetes, cerebral palsy, autism, or epilepsy.

The involvement of a credentialed school nurse can be pivotal for the student with PANS. The student will be at a distinct advantage that comes with having someone on the team, who by education, skill, and experience, recognizes the critical interplay of physiological systems that makes *any* academic achievement possible. Just as importantly, however, the nurse will also be the key figure on the team to recognize the ways in which an illness like PANS can thwart such development too.

Of course, the availability of school nurses varies dramatically from school to school. Even in areas where there are school nurses, schools may set up their IHCP systems very differently. For example, some have teams that also include a social worker and a school psychologist. In other school districts where school nurses serve large numbers of students, there may be 'health care assistants' who are not medically trained, *per se*, but serve as the "hands, eyes, and ears" for the credentialed school nurse at that school. She may be charged with such duties as administrating first aid, dispensing medications, verifying immunizations, and keeping the nurse apprised of current medical problems among students. In some instances, she or he might even do some procedures as gastrostomy/tube feeding of students. However, they are still considered to be "under the supervision" of the nurse, and not, by either training or certification, in a position to either make nursing decisions, or draw up health care plans.[10]

<u>Summary points of an IHCP</u> In an IHCP, the School Nurse and the team evaluate reports and information obtained from the physician, parents, and as much as possible, the student. They then determine what this information says in terms of what effects this illness has on the student. The rule of thumb for an IHCP is that the diagnosis does not drive the plan; rather, *the ways in which the illness or condition affects <u>this particular student</u> do.* Specifically, what can and should be done to address the student's needs that result from PANS? Listed below are a few aspects of what is typically included in an IHCP. They would, of course, address a wide range of illnesses, in addition to PANS.

- The student's medical diagnoses and summary of the student's health assessment data.
- The nursing diagnoses.
- Goals and actions related to the identified health problems/nursing diagnoses.
- Plans for handling emergency situations.
- Special considerations (equipment, medication, and so forth) for a student's participation in physical activities or sports (if applicable).
- Procedures to ensure safety and appropriate health services, which include school activities at school and on field trips.

Considerations for the Types and Ramifications of Assessments When Needed

Generally, the longer that the student has suffered from this condition, the greater the chances that she has also experienced impairment and regression of some kind. In order to clarify what the parameters of the student's abilities and disabilities are, testing may be warranted.

Regardless of whether the family requests psychoeducational testing from the school district or from outside sources, the unique parameters of a PANS diagnosis require that a number of considerations be taken into account.

- **Duration of the illness**. For some students, especially those who have been diagnosed and treated promptly, PANS may represent nothing more than a *blip on their medical and educational history*. Along with careful monitoring of their health status, and the carrying out of recommendations made through the IHCP, for example, teachers and parents would also simply observe for any changes.
- **Age.** The age of the student becomes a factor in that it is reflective of where he is developmentally. The fundamental assumption in learning is that a student continually scaffolds on new bits of

information, skills, and abilities, to what he's already mastered. For most children, this progression to higher developmental levels (in academics, self-help care, language skills, social skills, etc.) is fairly one directional.[11] Moreover, most, if not all of these disparate areas continue to develop. However, for the student with PANS, skills and abilities can actually regress, putting them at even more peril for jeopardizing a developmental base in which they scaffold on new knowledge and skills.

In particular, visual-perceptual difficulties, (a noted PANS symptom) can easily impede academic progress with younger students. This is because in most elementary classrooms, especially at the primary level, instruction is geared heavily towards the *visual sensory system* (the dominant sense for learning for most young children). If such difficulties were confirmed through testing, visual information could be supplanted or supported with auditory, tactile, or other kinds of information instead. By identifying and addressing such impairments, learning and skill development that is dependent on this type of processing would not continue to be compromised.

- **The health status of the student.** Test results may be compromised by the severity of symptoms during the time of the assessments. Perhaps the student hasn't slept well or eaten much during the last several weeks; perhaps he *appears* like he is complying with the examiner's requests for answers, but he is actually trying to tune out disturbing lights, sounds, anxieties, or something else. Perhaps the child has suffered a tiring and stressful trip to the testing site, and now has limited stamina to accurately demonstrate that which he is capable of. Alternatively, what if the student is tested during a "waning" period, which may illustrate his ability, but not the type of hindrances or limitations that would take place during a "waxing period?"
- **Testing as a transitional glimpse of the student's abilities.** Providers, student study team members, family members, and, as much as possible the student himself, should recognize the mere, *transitional glimpse* of his abilities that such testing provides. This speaks to the very erratic, unstable nature of the illness. If a student is able to complete testing, what are the plans to reassess him as he heals from the condition? If it is decided that no further testing will be needed in the future, how will the family/provider/school address the *meaning of test results* that at this *one point in time*, pointed to low functioning in numerous areas?
- **Financial resources of the family**, as well as accessibility to community or governmental resources, will offer advantages to allow for broader testing (or limit their procurement). In some situations, prior testing in psychoeducational testing, or testing in ancillary areas (such as vision, speech, or psychiatric/mental health), can assist the school toward more focused areas of exploration and treatment.
- **Testing as purposeful.** As the student's primary advocate, the parent *must* feel confident that the time, energy, expense, and potential stress surrounding getting this student to an evaluation is going to be worthwhile. Specifically, *how is the proposed testing or evaluation going to guide or provide services?* If the results of the evaluation indicate that the child has a diagnosis of Tourette Syndome or Oppositional Defiant Disorder (ODD), for example, what will such a diagnosis 'buy' in terms of actual help for the student? Moreover, how does the examiner situate the diagnosis in terms of the PANS illness? Is he clear in his understanding, and in his report (for example) that the ODD symptoms may not happen in all environments, and that they only *do* happen when the student is sick? Is he aware of the impermanent nature of these diagnoses related to PANS? Again, how is the evaluator tying test results to services and support for this young person?

This same litmus test should be considered in situations where parents are asked to have their child contribute to educational or other types of research. The parents should carefully balance the noble endeavor of expanding the knowledge base that the research can offer, with the potential risks and benefits for that student. Just as in medical research, where healing treatment to the patient has to be seen as the number one priority, (in other words, the generation of new theory must be secondary to the appropriate care of the patient), educational research, too, must identify ways in which the student's participation will result in (or at least, not impede) actual and specific remediation and/or other support for the child.

- **Inclusion of informal measures as beneficial too.** Finally, consider that there are a number of **non-standardized** or informal measures that can elicit information on how the student is functioning too. For example, at appointments:
  - What is the young person's appearance like?
  - What are his or her behaviors like, in terms of eye contact, unexpected movements, and verbal responses?
  - What was the student and parent experience of the trip getting over to the testing appointment? (Does the student remember? If it was dreadful, can he articulate why? How is his explanation different from that of his parent's?)
  - For a young student, can he draw a simple picture of himself, and what does it look like (compared to what his peers would draw)?
  - For an older student, how long does it take him to write down his list of classes? (Does he seem to be struggling to write, and what is the quality of the writing?)
  - Can the parent bring in samples of work that was completed pre-PANS and currently?
  - What is his speech and conversational levels like? (How does this compare to his same-aged peers?)
  - Can the young person give you *concrete* examples of the last time he 'hung out' with friends, and when he was actually invited by peers to functions, etc.? (How do these comments contrast to what the parents and others are observing and saying?)
  - If the teacher, provider, or other significant adult in the student's life can observe the student on the playground, in the classroom, or in other environments, how are this student's behaviors and interactions similar to or different from that of peers?
- **The Parent's Role in Safeguarding and 'Gatekeeping' Evaluation Results** Regardless of how one proceeds regarding the procurement of testing, it is important to keep in mind that the parents/guardians are the 'holders' of the records for their dependent minor child, and that the results of any medical, psychological, educational, or other evaluation are strictly **confidential**. As the minor child's legal guardian, they have the right to have access to testing results and reports about their child, to know exactly what is in their child's files, and to not allow access to others to see such documents.

  Moreover, if parents do not understand something that is written about their child (very often because reports can be written in a very technical fashion,[12] the parent must insist that there is someone at the evaluating facility who can and will 'translate' these results into understandable language. Moreover, if, for example, the parent requests testing for services for their child in US schools, they should know that the results and reports of such testing are typically kept in another area (outside of their student's regular academic 'Cume' folder). This means that regular education teachers and staff *will not* have access to this file.

  Furthermore, the parent *should not feel compelled* to automatically turn over each and every document pertaining to their child's testing results to schools or to other parties. Again, the litmus test for sharing such privileged information should be tied with *potential benefit to the student*, and relevance to what is being considered (such as interventions to address areas of weakness, etc.). In this regard, the parent might even choose to black out irrelevant (and sometimes erroneous) information, before submitting the report to third parties. They also might choose to limit *what topics or areas* that can be discussed with outside providers. For example, on forms indicating consents for the release of information, they might allow for a discussion of PANS symptoms to be held among providers and teachers, but not a discussion of *other* information (such as details regarding family dynamics, etc.). Alternatively, they might allow for this information to be exchanged, but only with a parent present.

In lengthily evaluations that include 'in-depth' medical and family histories, the evaluator and the parent should consider reviewing the "Background" sections of reports *before the final report* is drawn up- just to assure that what has been written is accurate. (Sometimes the evaluator might have misunderstood something in the intake screening where the background information about the child was elicited, or perhaps the evaluator included information from *other reports* that were misconstrued or inaccurate.) In any case, if parents read a report about their child that is inaccurate in any way, they have the right to ask the evaluator to make corrections. In cases where the report has not been modified to reflect what the parent believes is accurate or necessary, the parent can still write a note of retraction or disagreement to whoever did the evaluation, and request that this addendum be henceforth included with the report. Of course, the parent could, again, choose to submit the evaluation results with such information redacted (omitted or blacked out).

Finally, all parties must be careful about what is said in emails. This includes the relaying of such sensitive information as evaluation results, but it also includes any other information that should not be public knowledge. Even when such information is kept on dedicated computer servers, parents should consider asking *who has access* to these servers, and *how long the records are kept on these servers.* Hard copies (or paper copies) of sensitive reports are often considered to be the safest mode of document exchange.[13]

The Intrinsic Differences in *Perspective* among Students, Providers, and Parents

As families and schools pursue evaluations and referrals for their students, they must acknowledge the reality of, as well as the need for, hearing multiple and different perspectives on how PANS affects any one student. Very generally, and comparatively speaking, outside providers and school staff will report only a limited array of symptoms, in contrast to those who live with the child. The student, depending upon a number of factors that will be reviewed below, may also be far less circumspect in his awareness and/or articulation of how PANS affects him--and often even *less so* on how his illness (and resulting symptoms) affects others in his life. Moreover, parents of different families witnessing *the same intensity and frequency in behaviors and symptoms* may describe them very differently, in terms of debilitation, concern, and need. In these instances, varying perspectives will be influenced by a number of factors. A few of these may include social and cultural norms in the parent's community, social dynamics, other stressors within the family, and temperament of the parent reporting.

If the student has two parents, perspectives may also differ widely between the two, especially in situations where one parent is considered to be the 'primary care taker.' As with parenting any child with special needs, one parent is typically 'at a different point' than the other in terms of acceptance, involvement, and support of the ill child. In responding to inappropriate or unexpected behaviors of this child, for example, each parent will naturally be influenced by his or her *understanding* of the PANS mechanism itself, and how it can manifest in such behaviors. This level of understanding will often shape assumptions regarding *how much* their child's actions are attributable to *disease,* rather than to whatever the child's true 'character' or 'personality' might be. In turn, such insights regarding this 'why' of their child's behaviors, can serve to shape (or re-shape) 'the what,' regarding their *responses* to such behaviors. (Going even further, this knowledge might even serve to promote a sense of resolve and forgiveness on the part of others, who have dealt with the destructive turmoil associated with such troubling behaviors. This is especially true in families who have struggled with symptoms in a previously undiagnosed child for an extended time.)[14]

It must be assumed then, that there will be different perspectives gleaned from the patient, those closest to him, and adults who may see him intermittently. The following scenario is emblematic of a number of variables that can affect the depth and breadth of accurate information from a typical office visit- particularly one where the young person may be suffering from PANS.

Scenes from
~~The Doctor Visit~~

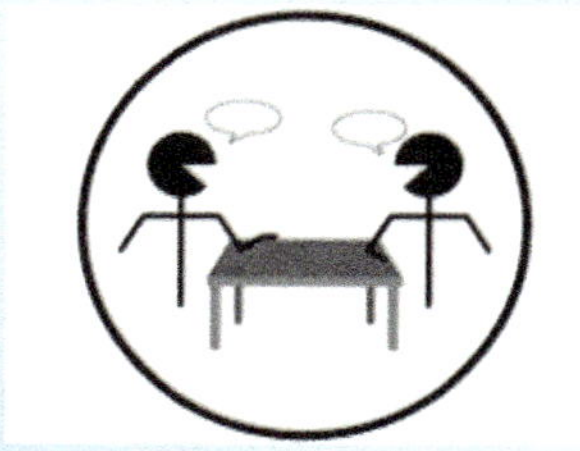

Doctor: *Oh, Ok...*
Mother: *Yes, Doctor- Well, going on to my 4th page of notes now...*
He's wetting the bed-
There's chronic spitting, barking sounds. No friends...

Later, after the parent has kindly been requested to "step outside for a few minutes."

Doctor: *So... How ya' doin?*
Sleepin' OK?
Hans: *Yeah.*
Doctor: *Hangin' out with friends?*
Hans: *Yeah.*
Doctor: *Anything bothering you?*
Hans: *Not really...*

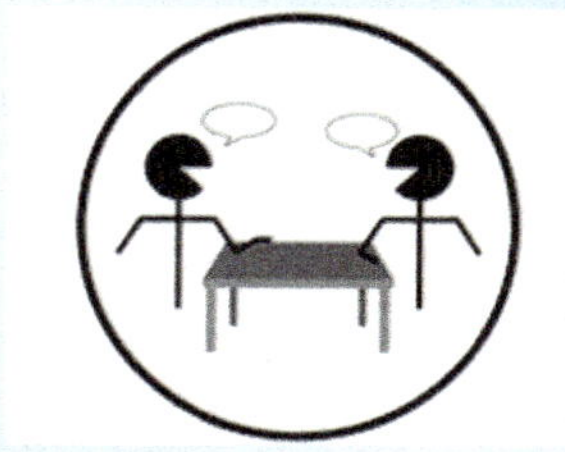

(Images courtesy of Reese Bretow, 2015)

- First of all, comments and feedback may be colored by general health status. Certainly, if the child is tired and ill, he may less predisposed to summon the energy to provide illuminating feedback. He may be irritable from the trip to the provider's office, and his attentional levels, regardless of his age, may be impaired. Timing of the appointment also figures prominently here. Unless providers are willing to visit in the early morning or late night hours at the home, for example, they should concede at the beginning that they will not be witnesses to the more extreme types of behavioral *Storms* and debilitation that the parent is probably seeing at home, usually at times of transition, where, for example, the children are going to bed or starting their day.
- Secondly, by PANS' very definition, some of this young person's cognitive processing abilities may be impaired at the time of the visit. As reviewed in Section I, PANS-related inflammation of the basal ganglia can result in slowed communication and efficiency amongst different parts of the brain.[15] Therefore, some may not process and respond to language and other cues as quickly as their peers might. Moreover, sickness behavior[16] and sleep difficulties may result in forgetfulness of events and behaviors that happened last week, or even that morning. Weakened visual perception can also result in uneven recall of events. At the same time, the *opposite* may be true. The young person may

present an appropriate and positive picture of what he is able to do *that afternoon*, but the office visit may lack glaring indications of debilitations seen by others two weeks ago, or three weeks hence.

- Thirdly, the child's responses may be conforming *first* to the dictates of whatever cultural and social expectations he has grown up with, before he devotes any such discourse to how he is *actually feeling*. Paradoxically, he may be 'doing his best' to respond to the provider's questions-- *at the expense of the purpose for the visit*. In this situation, any dialogue between the provider and the patient will become subject to both conscious and unconscious self-censure. Another variable at play here, is that for short periods of time, in new and unfamiliar environments, the child *will* often be able to rise to the occasion to appear at his best, *especially* if it is at a time of day that he typically has more energy and attention. Taken together then, if the provider asks, "How are you doing?" and, "Do you have friends?" the young person may register this to mean, "The doctor is having a polite conversation with me before the 'real' examination begins." Given this understanding, his appropriate responses would predictably be, "Yes, I am fine. And yes, I hang out with friends all the time." In this way, it is important to recognize that the mandate and the constraints of the discourse will be very different for the patient, than it is for the parent and/or the provider.

Let us take a moment to carry this particular aspect of *Provider dialogues* further. The following comments shed light on how important it is for such interviews to be handled very carefully by both providers and adult family members.

> ..."*I just got so tired and resentful of dragging him to another doctor who basically wanted a dog and pony show--right there in the office--of how crazy (my son) was so he could finally be convinced that what I was saying was real, and we could get help! It was really humiliating for Hans*[17] ... *I couldn't stand it. I was saying stuff about (Hans) that I knew he didn't want anybody to know about... (The doctor) would ask me questions about him--when he was right there in the room! And then he'd ask Hans, "Is this true?" Yeah! Like every kid wants strangers to know that he still wets the bed and that he spits all over! What an idiot! It was just so sad, because (Hans) was just trying to do everything he could to 'keep it together' until the appointment was over. After that last time, I swore I'd never do* that *to him again.*"[18]

This unfortunate experience points to the importance of assuring that parents and other adults (or even interviewed siblings, or others) are offered opportunities *to speak alone with the provider* (either during the appointment or earlier/later on the phone). This will serve to both elicit their valuable perspective, and to safeguard, validate, and honor the unique perspective, experience, and feelings of all concerned.

- Fourth, numerous studies, as well as commonly acknowledged observations on males and females, show how there are differences in the quantity and quality of verbal disclosures made, based on gender differences alone. Cognitive strengths favor females in the areas of language facility and social skills in general (longer length of utterances, better at reading character and social cues, better grammar and vocabulary, better perception of sounds, longer attention span, increased use of eye contact, etc.[19] [20] Moreover, there will again be cultural and social mandates specific to males and females, that consciously (and unconsciously) influence comfort levels related to sensitive disclosures. For boys and young men, especially, this may mean that they will be more guarded about disclosing potentially embarrassing or unflattering symptoms (such as bedwetting or having frequent meltdowns).[21]
- Fifth, a young person's developmental stage, as typically reflected by age, (and affected by the regression that can occur with PANS) will figure prominently in such discourse. In terms of depth and breadth of language of course, but also in terms of memory and reasoning ability. For it is these

variables that will help determine how PANS and all of its related interventions and treatments (medications, supplements, behavioral therapies, etc.) *are understood* to be affecting them. Generally, the older students are, for example, the better they will remember the multiple variations of their *feeling well* (or well enough), before the onset of PANS symptoms. Moreover, they will also have the language skills and life experiences to know (and to separate) this *current state of health and well-being*, from what their *normal* states are. At the same time, for long term sufferers who have had an early onset of PANS especially, their (relative) lack of memories, experiences, reasoning ability, and language skills may combine to acutely, and negatively, shape their understandings and assumptions of what their current experience is, and how it is situated within the larger scope of what life is *supposed to be* like.

- And last, but not least, in certain instances, is important to consider the possibility that the young person may have now decided to act on an inner resolve (consciously or unconsciously) to say as little as possible to new providers---*lest he need to come back.*

As in the stories of the young adult survivors interviewed,[22] many patients with PANS made long, difficult journeys to see a number of different providers before they were finally and correctly diagnosed with PANS. Until that time, however, most perceived little to no difference in their *actual comfort* as a result of these visits. At worse, these appointments meant even more traveling and medical interventions, such as painful blood draws, medications, and other unpleasant treatments. Over time, experience had taught them then, that such visits are difficult at best, and painful at worst. Better to avoid the whole thing and stay home...

The Notion of Least Restrictive Environment (LRE) and PANS

Specifically, what does the directive of *Least Restrictive Environment* mean for the student with PANS, who may be off the *fully-included-regular-education-track* for uncertain periods of time?

When parents consider asking their school district to provide any kind of "Special Services" or other types of interventions for their child, they may have only a generalized idea of what this means. Some may, in fact, lump any kind of help with 'special education,' and believe that if their child receives help, it would take place in a separate setting for all or part of the day. They may worry that if their child requires special education, for example, that access to a regular education curriculum may be threatened. However, in practice, services, accommodations (such as extra time on tests), and type and number of minutes of special education provided to students vary widely among students needing help. A brief discussion and examples of the concept of Least Restrictive Environment will shed light on just how individualized and varied such services really are, and of course, must be.

Least Restrictive Environment concerns the importance of educating students with disabilities in regular education or **mainstreamed** classes first (with appropriate aids and supports where needed), *before* it is recommended that they be transferred to more restrictive (or separate) learning environments. It is intended to provide all students with opportunities for learning, to the extent that they are able. It concerns the importance of providing a fifth grade student with a reading disability, for example, the same opportunity as his peers to have access to a fifth grade curriculum, including grade level math and history, etc. However, it also implicitly addresses the need for students to have access to the **non-academic** aspects of a mainstreamed learning environment too. This includes the social, physical, and extracurricular opportunities that public education provides, such as field trips, sports activity, and dances.

At the same time, the mandate of Least Restrictive Environment requires that if a student is placed in, for example, a regular education classroom, that it is expected that the student will obtain *clear benefit from that placement*. Certainly, it is not the intent of this mandate to allow students to flounder in educational placements that they are not able to receive educational benefit from.

A key concept here is to examine the *intensity* and *frequency* of any symptoms and behaviors that compromise learning and participation. These can include such things as incompletion of work and non-participation in activities, but it can also include verbal and physical outbursts (including reactivity to sensory input or OCD triggers), lethargy, extreme inattentiveness, etc. When this student is showing indications that full participation is being compromised, an IEP or 504 meeting is warranted to reassess levels of need and support. These meetings should include the credentialed school nurse, and outside mental healthcare professionals as needed. Examples of levels and types of support are included in the chart below.

Example of a Continuum of Alternative Placements

Least Restrictive Environment

- Implementation of an Individualized Health Care Plan (IHCP), whereby the student is allowed to take his own PANS- related medications at lunchtime (on campus or on fieldtrips), and where the staff notifies parent if there is an outbreak of an infection (i.e. Strep) in the school.
- An IHCP and a 504, whereby a nurse may dispense medications at lunch time to the student, and whereby on field trip, either she or a designated individual under her supervision is responsible to dispense PANS medications.
- IHCP and/or 504 accommodations -such as extra time on tests, etc.- with check ins by a 504 Coordinator with student and teachers several times a month)
- IHCP and the following:
- Regular education with weekly monitoring from a special ed. provider.
- Regular education with daily consultation from a special ed. provider.
- Regular education with special education services and supports included in that setting, which are aligned with the general curriculum utilizing such strategies as:
  - Flexible groupings among students.
  - "Universally"-designed curriculum to serve students' unique learning needs.
  - Peer tutoring, cooperative learning in small groups.
  - Team teaching with 2 teachers with different expertise.

More Restrictive Environment

- Regular education, with special education services provided *for part of the day* in a resource room or a special ed. classroom
- Regular education with home/ hospital instruction provided by a certificated teacher in general education (or if in middle or high school, teachers in such subject areas (such as Math, etc.) provided for part of the day with special ed. consultation (to all teachers, student, and/or parent on a weekly basis.
- Instruction in regular education and specialty subjects provided at the student's home for most of the day (or week), with participation in some mainstreamed general education classes at school *for part of the day* (or week). Special Ed. consultation on a weekly or daily basis.
- Self-contained special education classroom.
- Special day school (outside the school environment).
- Residential School facility (offering ranges of regular/special ed.)
- Special Ed. in most areas of instruction at home or in the hospital.
- Home or Hospital instruction (with limited or highly variable quantities and areas of instruction), with little access to peers/outside activity.

Most Restrictive Environment

Considerations Regarding the Degree and Type of Support Needed

Both families *and* school communities will need support as they strive to help their students who struggle with PANS. Part of this support will include **advocacy**. The notion of advocacy often denotes an individual who is paid to speak assertively and knowledgeable on behalf of the student. However, as with other areas associated with this paradigm-changing condition, there will be a range of advocacy services that will be appropriate (or even necessary), as the symptoms of the illness play out in the educational setting.

At the same time, it is important for *both* the teacher and family to know what options are available, should the illness remain or progress, and concerns start to heighten. Awareness of what is done for other students in similar situations, can also serve to relieve some of the worry that comes with not knowing what's within the 'acceptable parameters of service' for this student. At a minimum, it may be helpful to look at some of the websites that are listed in the reference section, and referred to in other areas of this book. Many of these will outline related systems, programs, and services. Generally speaking, it is best for both families and teachers to seek out advice and support from 'within' before bringing in 'outsiders,' (who can sometimes be seen as the more adversarial 'big guns'). For example, the constructive involvement of those considered to be 'non-teaching staff' (such as School nurses, School Social Workers, counselors, and School Psychologists, etc.) can help avert potential pitfalls and frustration, as the educational process continues to unfold.

Of course, the most ideal situation is where the parent and the teacher(s) work together to address the needs of the student, without bringing in the administration, district level staff, or 'outsiders' to resolve issues and delegate tasks. If a special education teacher is being sought out to serve as the caseworker and liaison between the school parent and student, it behooves both the parent and the teacher(s) to be a team. An important concept for all to remember is, that as much as possible, and for as long as possible; give each other the benefit of the doubt, and assume that each is doing the best she or he can under the circumstances. The building up of trust and goodwill among the key people in the student's life can make a huge difference in educational planning and outcomes later on.

On this theme, I am reminded of how a friend spoke of how, on the morning of her wedding, her mother came into her room and summoned her over to sit down on the bed. "Oh Dear," my friend thought as she mentally began to dread what the *pre-wedding advice* might be. Undeterred by her daughter's worried frown, Mrs. Scott began. "Honey, I really only have one piece of advice to give you on your wedding day." She took a serious pause, braced herself, and then spilled it out- "Even if you don't *like* your mother-in-law, LIKE your mother-in-law." "Well..." she concluded, "That's it." And she walked out and poured herself a pre-wedding whisky.

It's a little like that with teachers and parents, especially when both are so directly and pivotally involved in the life of a student with such needs as PANS. As good faith gestures, parents can bring the teacher the odd latte, or convey kind words of acknowledgement for ideas and interventions that parents find to be helpful. Teachers can show parents that they have investigated PANS, by going on the internet, or by looking at other resources. The accumulation of small words of appreciation, smiles, and acknowledgements of the things *that are going right,* can go a long way to foster positive and effective collaboration- so needed in the educational care of this student.

<u>*When there appears to be a 'mismatch' between expectations and delivery of services,*</u>[23] the parent should consider the following obstacles that may, in fact, be at play:

- The teacher may not really have the expertise or support to accommodate the student, but feels that somehow she *should* be knowledgeable and capable of doing what is needed, and is reluctant to ask for help out of fear of appearing incompetent.
- The teacher does not have the expertise or support to accommodate the student, but is striving to do her best to help the student by asking other staff for advice in the interim.
- The teacher does not have the expertise or support to help the student, and the administration and interpersonal dynamics at the school (and school district) do not foster an environment where requests for teacher training and mentoring are supported and encouraged. Also, she may

be aware that support services, such as school nursing, counseling, and assistive technology, take a long time to secure, are "too expensive," or are simply unavailable.

- The teacher *does* have the expertise, and at least minimal amounts of support allotted to help the student (like a class assistant), but education is still compromised because of other factors, including the needs of other students in the class, personality and expertise of assigned paraprofessionals, and communication difficulties with the special education teacher and/or other case workers or counselors.
- The special education teachers (in particular) may be relegated to portables or other small rooms (away from the 'regular education' classrooms) and/or they may not be acknowledged/ integrated/supported by other school staff, as being "one of them." As wonderful and skilled as the individual teacher may be with her students, the parent should be cognizant of the degree to which this teacher has the respect and voice amongst her peers, as this, by extension, can affect the nature of services provided to her students, especially outside of that classroom.
  In this same regard, whereas many teachers (in both regular and special education) will be kind and helpful to their students, their efforts may be thwarted by their administration's lack of proactivity when it comes to serving students with any kind of special learning needs.

Broadening the Notion of Support and Advocacy

As the needs of the student evolve, and in some cases, become more demanding, varying levels of support may be considered. Following is a discussion of four types of support and advocacy that families and educators may find useful. Regardless of the severity of the situation though, keep in mind that in many areas, there is access to a number of advocacy groups that can usually be reached by phone or on the internet. State agencies, parent groups, and other (primarily) nonprofit groups run many such organizations, designed to provide counseling to those wishing to clarify aspects of obtaining special education and services in their area. Moreover, many of these agencies are free or at low cost. Aside from such groups dedicated to helping students with special needs (in general), there are advocacy groups addressed to issues *specific to PANS* symptoms as well, and some of these are listed in the resource section.

1. *Parental and Teacher Awareness of the Prevailing Laws and Procedures Surrounding Services and Services.* Along with knowing the parameters of the effect the illness is having on the student's progress, an awareness of some of the main laws surrounding IEPS, accommodations, and special education, can be very useful. This information can be obtained by either looking up the information on line, by asking for a copy of such information at the school,[24] or by contacting county, state, or national agencies. Other options that are at no cost or low cost are parent advisory boards dealing with student rights in special education, and citizen rights as an individual with disabilities.

In the US, it is helpful to know some basic tenets of legislation, such as *Federal Laws regarding special education prevail in each state.* Moreover, one should know that in actuality, there is a very broad range of acceptable services and accommodations that student study teams are empowered to endorse. Although it may not be acknowledged openly, consider the possibility that personnel at the school or district may be unaware of the latest laws. This is why it is so important for the parent and the teacher to be either aware of such information themselves, or at least, know where they can get easy access to such information.

2. *Parental and/or Teacher Awareness of Services and Accommodations That Are Considered to Be "Acceptable and Appropriate."* Both parents and school staff may be actually unaware of what is

truly considered *'acceptable and appropriate'* when it comes to serving our students with PANS. As a result, attendees at meetings may deny services like home/hospital schooling because in truth, they may not feel empowered or confident that they *can allow* for such services. With regard to advocating for modifications and services, information from the *pandasnetwork.org* website or other articles pertaining to PANS and education can be very helpful and validating. This information is important to have access to at planning meetings. At the same time, however, it is always a good idea to pass copies along to key members of the team to study *in advance* of these meetings too. Such articles will provide written (and therefore compelling) documentation that certain accommodations, modifications, and services *are* acknowledged by specialists in the PANS field- *to be appropriate and necessary* to the educational goals of a child with this condition. This documentation, in turn, will help bolster the *decision-makers'* confidence and resolve that the services really are essential to this child. As a result, when they need to answer to *their* superiors, they will have something in writing to support this need for services. (Of course, these would supplement the letters of need coming from the child's medical providers and parents too.)

3. *The Involvement of Significant Others* At educational meetings, the inclusion of outside providers (such as therapists, religious leaders, family members, and trusted friends) can serve as advocates, and just as importantly, provide moral support for parents and the student. Their very presence at these meetings can make a difference in terms of its tone and direction. This is true, even if they say nothing. Their presence can often serve to 'even up' the power balance at the meeting. These attendees also act as witnesses to what is being said. Mostly though, these others act as visual forms of support to the parent who is usually speaking as the student's primary advocate. For clearly, it can often be intimidating for a parent to sit amongst a group of people who have pivotal decision-making roles, that will not only affect her or his child, but by extension, their entire family.

4. *If Circumstances Come To Pass where Outside (Professional) Advocacy Is Needed,* the following considerations may help guide in the selection of an advocate:

The key towards finding a professional educational advocate is *experience, experience, experience.* A special education, administrative, neuropsychological, and/or legal background is very helpful in this regard, as well. A good 'seasoned' advocate will know current changes in special education law, and of its related implications on student services and interventions. She will also be aware of potential hurdles surrounding specific school district policies and personnel. Last, but not least, she (or he) will have the temperament, social skills, and language finesse to *both* facilitate a positive, collaborative working relationship with the school, *and* tactfully 'draw the line,' such as demanding more for the student. Referrals from other parents or parent advisory boards dealing with student rights and procedural safeguards in special education can be extremely helpful in this regard.

In a similar vein, should teachers or other staff members feel that they need help and advocacy outside the hierarchy of the school district, they might consider contacting their union, teacher specialty organizations (such as those specializing in their subject matter), or other agencies that may provide assistance.

And Finally... Journeying Down the Road Less Traveled: Lessons From Harriet Tubman

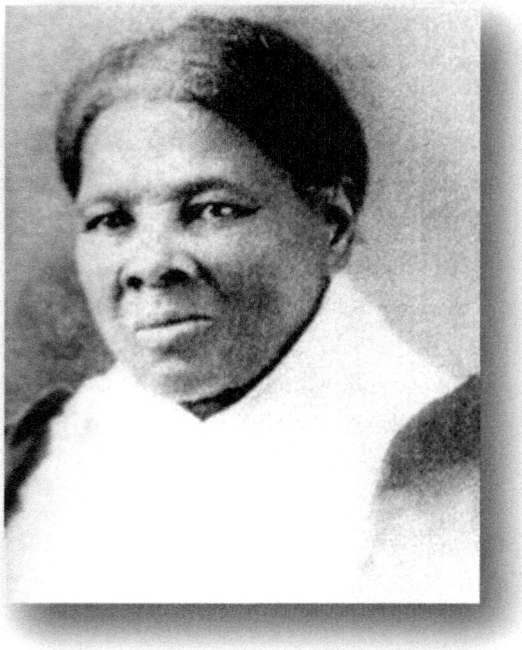

Harriet Tubman (c. 1822-1913)[25]
"Just Keep Going"

Harriet Tubman may never have actually uttered those famed sentiments that are so often attributed to her... "If you're hungry you keep going, if you're tired, you keep going, if you're sick, you just keep going, etc.." However, she did point out that as the 'Conductor' of the *Underground Railroad,* where she ferried escaped slaves from the pre-Civil War South to freedom in Canada, she never lost a passenger... not once in 19 harrowing trips. So, in fact, we can assume that these rescued men, women, children, and even infants, did indeed "just keep going." This, despite the fact that they were escaping on foot, at night, in the bitter cold of winter... over impossibly long expanses of the North American eastern seaboard. Worse, Harriet Tubman made these journeys knowing that at any time, she could be instantly incapacitated from 'drop' seizures (resulting from a severe head assault with a metal weight that she had suffered as a teen).

When families have a child touched by PANS, there is so much at stake. Despite a strong desire for their child to resume to a pre-PANS educational curriculum as soon as possible, physical and psychological concerns are always at the forefront of their worries. At PANS' worst manifestations, parents may rightfully feel grateful and successful if *everyone in the family is still alive at the end of the day*. Working up from that very minimal, but critical bar, it is not impossible, though, to take steps, albeit tiny ones, towards going forward on the academic escalator too.

As will be illustrated more fully in Section VI, there are a number of ways that academic learning can be woven into the student's day to bolster whatever capacities that are still functioning. Perhaps the student can listen to a home/hospital teacher or parent read a chapter of a school book for fifteen minutes a day. Often, there will be times during the day that these students will be calmer or more focused, such as the afternoon or evening. Perhaps during these times, they can dictate a few sentences of homework or responses to test questions into an *iphone,* and the parent can send the voice clip on to the class teacher. Perhaps they cannot attend the whole school day, but they do have the stamina to attend during the afternoon, etc. The point is to take a page from Ms. Tubman and to just keep going forward- doing as much as the student is reasonably capable of, considering his present limitations. He may not yet be back to the level of quality and quantity of academic work that he was doing prior to PANS. Still, loved ones and educators should feel confident that even 30% of the level of prior work can be recognized as a valiant success, if it furthers any academic progress. Consider too, that academic progress also includes progress and development in social skills and other areas- (that don't necessarily involve reading, writing, or arithmetic).

The process of participating in, and negotiating a school environment for even *part of the day*, if the child is well enough, has value too. As the student transitions from illness to wellness, even small amounts of instruction and participation in academic and social activity will minimize the extent of educational repercussions later on. For, whether it is addressing medical, psychological, or educational manifestations of this illness, loved ones and providers will agree with Ms. Tubman- that there is no going back, *only forward*. Taking a page from Ms. Tubman then, deliverance comes from looking at the end goal, and breaking it down into tiny, but attainable steps.

As we take steps then to obtain help for students with PANS, what can we expect from the entity in which we regularly entrust the care of children for most of their productive day? Section IV will familiarize the reader with an example of one country's agreed-upon parameters, regarding what is considered to be 'accepted and appropriate care' for students with disabling conditions.

Notes

[1] Candelaria Greene, J. F. (2015) Unpublished survey of family members, providers, and survivors of PANS regarding PANS and Education, collected as UC Berkeley Visiting Researcher Scholar (2013-2015), Berkeley, California.

[2] Larson, K., Russ, S., Kahn, R. S., & Halfon, N. (2007) Patterns of Comorbidity, Functioning, and Service Use for US Children with ADHD. Pediatrics.

[3] Similarly, students with Down Syndrome (Trisomy 21) also have a much higher incidence of comormid conditions than their non-affected peers, such as congenital cardiac and gastrointestinal tract conditions. (Ram G., Chinen, J. (2011) Infections and immunodeficiency in Down syndrome. Clinical and Experimental Immunology. 2011;164(1):9-16. These students may also have Atlantoaxial Instability (a misalignment of the top two vertebrae of the neck). Still, many students with Trisomy 21 tend to be served primarily for an intellectual disability, and often (but not always) a speech and language impairment. Typically, students with Trisomy 21 are not served in the school setting for impairment in the areas of psychiatric or behavioral disorders. In contrast, as parents and special educators reported, students with PANS were typically receiving services to accommodate for multiple impairments. These took place both inside and outside of the school setting (Candelaria Greene, 2015).

[4] Certainly, *all students,* including students who are receiving school services for identified impairments, including health conditions, will experience significant fluctuations in the course of their education- physically, socially, psychologically, motorically, etc. Moreover, it is not uncommon to see both positive and negative changes that can affect academic progress. However, the majority of these students, even in special education classrooms, will not experience the ***substantial*** and ***radical*** waxing of symptoms and abilities, as students with PANS do. (Candelaria Greene, J. F., 2015).

[5] (Which is increasing in availability, but still often difficult to find across the US, and in other countries).

[6] pandasnetwork.org PANDAS/PANS Statistics 2014-2015http://pandasnetwork.org/wp-content/uploads/2014/11/Statistics-PANDAS-Network.pdf (retrieved April 2015).

[7] Candelaria Greene, J. F. (2015).

[8] (Though not codified under federal law.)

[9] *Primary Disabling Condition* (US) refers to the primary identifier that warrants special education or other services in schools. Examples of this include *Other Health Impairment* (which includes PANS), or *Specific Learning Disability.*

[10] For their thoughtful comments on this subject, the author wishes to thank Amy Joy Fishman Smith NP, Celine Forte RN of Smithfield School District, Rhode Island, and Jodi Biskup RN and Alison Angell of Alameda Unified School District, California (Feb/March 2015).

[11] Such growth is also broad in scope, in that in most individuals, most areas of function rise together (i.e. language skills, reasoning, gross motor skills, etc.).

[12] Often to relate to both the style and practice of other providers, whom they may be sending reports too.

[13] For these reasons, it is also prudent to avoid sending highly sensitive information by email, even amongst day-to-day communications with the teacher.

[14] As noted by respondents' comments (Candelaria Greene, 2015).

[15] Murphy, T. K., Patel, P. D., McGuire, J. F., Kennel, A., Mutch, P. J., Parker-Athill, E. C., Hanks, C. E., Lewin, A. B., Storch, E. A., Toufexi, M. D., Dadlani, G. H., & Rodriguez, C.A. (2015). Characterization of the Pediatric Acute-Onset Neuropsychiatric Syndrome Phenotype Journal of Child and Adolescent Psychopharmacology. February 2015, 25(1): 14-25. doi:10.1089/cap.2014.0062.

[16] Ibid.

[17] Candelaria Greene, J. F. (2015). "Hans" is a fictional name as are other names of interviewees, unless stated otherwise.

[18] Candelaria Greene, J. F. (2015) (H. R. notes).

[19] Moir, A.,& Jessel, D. (1991) Brain Sex: The Real Difference Between Men and Women. Carol Publishing/Lyle Stuart New York.

[20] Howard, P. (2000) The Owner's Manual for the Brain: Everyday applications from mind-brain research, 2nd edition. Austin, TX: Bard Press p 216-234.

[21] Candelaria Greene, (2015).

[22] Ibid.

[23] (Note how none of this really has anything to do with traits, qualities, or abilities of the parent or child in question.)

[24] In the US, a copy of what is called *Procedural Safeguards* describes such information, and by law it should be available at all public schools.

[25] (Photo credit https://commons.wikimedia.org/wiki/File:Harriet-Tubman-248x300.jpg) with thanks to Graphic Designer Reese Bretow, 2015).

Section IV

AN OVERVIEW OF LEGISTLATION RELATED TO SPECIAL EDUCATION AND SERVICES (US): What This Means for Students with PANS

A Societal Commitment to Fair Access to Educational Opportunities

'School' constitutes a major part of a student's day, and in most countries, a major part of one's childhood and adolescence. It is where young people *go off to* each day for their 'work.' For most youth today, being a 'student' truly *is* their career. School provides them with knowledge and skills, but it also gives them critical feedback, both positive and negative, on the degree to which they are *successfully* functioning - academically, socially, and motorically, etc. Such judgments are typically made in comparison with their same aged peers.

These types of feedback, in turn, play a critical and pivotal role in determining what students' *educational choices and opportunities* will be as they progress through the grades. Years later, when the student finally steps off the scholastic escalator that opens up into the adult world of functional independence and employment, it will be *that feedback* that will have largely shaped the student's experience, preparedness, and outcomes. Very often, this academic experience and preparedness is often the litmus test of what is regarded as a 'good education.' Yet, *the degree* to which a young person can learn and gain from this 'good education' will depend, not only on the student herself, but on the degree to which she has had access to it.

Access can be jeopardized for a number of reasons, including everything from logistical constraints to student malnutrition, weak family or community support, or an established disabling condition such as deafness. In the case of a student with PANS, access to an education that is "free and appropriate" can be clearly thwarted by the debilitating symptoms of the illness itself. Moreover, the educational experience of this student *will* be jeopardized, unless of course, help is provided along the way. Such needed assistance should be designed to assure a fair access to a good learning environment, and as reasonably as possible- a 'level playing field,' where each and every student is offered effective opportunities to learn, and, if needed, the additional support to succeed.

In reading the overview of the educational laws below, one quickly will become cognizant of how (US) legislation *does* acknowledge conditions (such as PANS) as being, at the very least, *potentially* disabling. In turn, such acknowledgement opens the door to related assessments, accommodations, and other services, such as special education, etc.

Legislation Affecting Students with Disabilities

As with any other crisis or emergency, it is helpful for *all involved* to be familiar with, at least, the basic tenets of legislation that are designed to help students, should they suffer disabilities. These include disabilities that may be temporary in nature, such as PANS. Practically speaking, knowledge of one's local and national educational safety nets can both facilitate the appropriate delivery of educational services, and reduce the uncertainty and frustration often associated with obtaining help for students with disabilities.

In the United States, for example, most of the special education and educational accommodations and services stem from major acts of legislation such as **Section 504** and **IDEA**. These laws mirror similar frameworks found in various school districts, states, and other countries too. Although US law is presented as an example here, *the point is solely to become familiar with one's own sets of rules that regulate one's school's policies.* In most cases, this information can easily be obtained by visiting related websites at the state level (in the US), or by contacting local educational agencies in their home cities or countries. Nonprofit agencies, serving disabled populations in general, and students with disabilities in particular, are also good sources, especially if a person wants to speak to an expert one-on-one about the application of current laws as they pertain to a specific student or situation.

Section 504 and ADA

In 1977, **Section 504 of the <u>Rehabilitation Act of 1973</u>**[1] was enacted to prohibit discrimination against individuals with disabilities. This is largely regarded as the first civil-rights statute for people with disabilities. Within this scope, it was designed to ensure that all students with a disability have equal *access* to an education. Essentially, Section 504 prohibits discrimination against persons with a disability in *any program receiving federal financial assistance.*

Section 504 is broadly defined. Consider the breadth and depth of 504's parameters: It recognizes a person with a disability as anyone who has "a physical or mental impairment, has a record of such an impairment, or is regarded as having such an impairment, which substantially limits one or more **major life activities**, such as caring for one's self, performing manual tasks, walking, seeing, hearing, speaking, breathing, learning, working, sleeping, standing, lifting, reading, concentrating, thinking, communicating, helping, eating, bending, or operation of a bodily function."[2] Examples of students who are typically served under Section 504 include those with "asthma, allergies, and chemical sensitivities, mobility issues or physical disabilities, limited eyesight or hearing, cancer, Depression, Anxiety (or other mental health conditions), Attention Deficit Disorder (ADD)/Attention Deficit Hyperactivity Disorder (ADHD), Dyslexia and diabetes, and those who are medically fragile..." Moreover, *major life activities* can also include bodily functions, such as "functions of the immune system, normal cell growth, digestive, bowel, bladder, neurological, brain, respiratory, circulatory, endocrine, and reproductive functions."[3]

It may surprise the reader to discover that Section 504 does not fall under *Education Law*, but rather, *Civil Rights Law*. That said, it still includes provisions for identifying and referring potential students with suspected disabilities (such as *Child Find*), evaluations to determine disabilities, and the development of a 504 Plan, sometimes called an **Individual Accommodation Plan (IAP)**.

In the case of a student with symptomatology of PANS, it would be well under the auspices of a 504, for example, to make a referral to providers (working for the school district) or *outside providers* (practitioners in the community) to determine the nature and extent of symptoms, and to address the educational repercussions of such symptoms. Moreover, this law provides for such services to occur whether a diagnosis of PANS had been made yet, or not.

<u>Specific Provisions of Section 504 and Title II</u>

Technically, **Section 504** applies to *the recipients of grants or monies* from the federal government, and **Title II** applies only to *public entities* (such as public schools and colleges). Sometimes, schools will be both a public entity, and also a recipient of federal monies. In these cases, the institution will be covered by both laws. Both of these laws protect all participants in the program, <u>including students, parents, and employees</u>, from discrimination. Moreover, these laws cover *all of the programs* of a school or college, including academic, extracurricular, and athletic functions. They include those that occur off campus too (such as participation on field trips or graduation ceremonies). Lastly, under **both** Section 504 and Title II of the Americans with Disabilities Act, it is unlawful to *harass people in 'covered entities'* because of their disabilities.[4]

<u>Modifications, Accommodations, Related Aids, and Services under 504</u>

Commonly used **modifications** and **accommodations** under 504 include building accessibility (such as the use of elevators if a child is in a wheelchair), classroom accommodations (such as extra time on tests), or curriculum modifications (such as the use of Braille instead of the use of a printed only textbooks). Other examples include: getting one's medication during the school day, modified participation in gym or adaptive physical education, use of a computer or other needed technology, use of a recording device or calculator, taking tests in quiet locations, receiving a '**Behavior Intervention Plan**,' getting the assistance of a para-professional, guidance counselor, or social worker, and having a modified classroom schedule. (Also see related discussion on Modifications and Accommodations in the appendix.)

Related aids and **services** provided under Section 504 include school health services, transportation, counseling, speech and language services, audiology services, physical and occupational therapy services, orientation and mobility services, and counseling services.[5] [6] They also can include environmental, instructional, and behavioral accommodations, as well as provisions for a modified schedule, grading system, or curriculum.

The Americans with Disabilities Act (1990), commonly referred to as **ADA**, was legislation enacted to prohibit discrimination against persons with a disability in any program receiving federal financial assistance. ADA disabilities include both mental and physical medical conditions. One might hear of buildings or bathroom facilities that are "**ADA compliant**," meaning that they have been designed, or modified, to ensure greater access to all- including those with disabilities. An obvious example of this is *wheelchair accessibility* through the use of ramps and elevators.

In terms of serving individuals with PANS, it is important to know that these conditions don't necessarily need to be *severe* or *permanent* to be considered a "disability." Moreover, ADA acknowledged that certain mental or physical health conditions (such as diabetes, for example) *could* be covered disabilities, depending upon what the individual's symptoms are in the *absence* of "**mitigating measures**," such as medication, assistive devices, therapy, or other means of restoring function during an "active episode" of a health condition that is considered episodic."[7]

The **Americans with Disabilities Amendments Act of 2008** broadened the meaning of "disabled student" under Section 504. For example, the term "physical or mental impairment" would no longer be limited to any *specific* diseases or categories of medical conditions. Furthermore, a simple comparison with a student's *non-disabled age/grade peers* could suffice when determining whether an impairment was said to "substantially limit a major life activity" for the student.

The term "*major life activities*" would now be interpreted more broadly as well, to include most activities that are considered to be important in a school-aged student's daily life. Moreover, the fact that the impairment only limited one major life activity was sufficient enough to obtain help; it did not need to necessarily affect several domains of functioning (such as poor motor skills and weak intellectual ability). Next, the consideration of "Mitigating Measures," discussed earlier, was now completely disregarded when determining whether a student's impairment constituted a disability under Section 504 or ADA.

Of particular relevance to many students with PANS, is clear language regarding the expectation that there will be evaluations to rule out *even a temporary impairment* as a disability. In this case, 'temporary' is meant to have an actual or expected duration of six months or less. Moreover, this same legislation expressly concerns conditions that are also *episodic in nature,* or in *remission*. The primary consideration here is focused squarely on the extent to which the condition *limits a major life activity* for the student.

Individuals with Disabilities Education Act (IDEA)

In 1975, US Public Law 94-142, (also called the **Education for All Handicapped Children Act**) was legislated to assure that "all children with disabilities have available to them ... a free appropriate public education, which emphasizes Special Education and related services designed to meet their unique needs." This law was designed to ensure that the "rights of children with disabilities and their parents ... are protected," and that states and localities were assisted to provide for the education of all children with disabilities. A "free and appropriate education"[8] (FAPE) falls under IDEA and the Rehabilitation Act.

Later codified as the **Individuals with Disabilities Education Act (IDEA)**, federal legislation addressed **how** states and public agencies provided early intervention, special education, and related services to students with disabilities. IDEA specifically defines a **disabling condition** as one that *adversely affects* educational performance, and cites the following categories of disability:

- Autism
- Deaf-Blindness
- Deafness
- Developmental Delay
- Emotional Disturbance
- Hearing Impairment
- Intellectual Disability
- Multiple Disabilities
- ***Other Health Impairment (OHI)*** (which PANS would fall under)
- Specific Learning Disability
- Speech or Language Impairment

- Traumatic Brain Injury (TBI), and
- Visual Impairment (including blindness)[9]

Other Health Impairment (OHI) and PANS

Of special importance to students with PANS, let's pause to take a closer look at the definition of *Other Health Impairment,* one of the specific categories of disability that warrants special education, and then highlight some of its implications:

> "***Other Health Impairment*** *means having limited strength, vitality, or alertness, including a heightened alertness to environmental stimuli, that results in limited alertness with respect to the educational environment, that: i. Is due to chronic or acute health problems such as asthma, attention deficit disorder or attention deficit hyperactivity disorder, diabetes, epilepsy, a heart condition, hemophilia, lead poisoning, leukemia, nephritis, rheumatic fever, sickle cell anemia, and Tourette's syndrome; and (ii) Adversely affects a child's educational performance."*[10]

Inherent in its definition OHI does the following:

- Acknowledges disabling conditions (such as PANS) that are chronic, but not necessarily permanent.
- Directly recognizes that the symptoms of the *illness* are the source of the academic difficulties.
- Acknowledges that substantial variations in function (across the domains) can exist, and that, just as importantly, also exist within that particular student (i.e. fluctuations in achievement and abilities).

It is possible, as is the case with other students who have an IEP, that some students with PANS may also be served for other disabilities too (such as *'Specific Learning Disability'* or *'Speech and Language' Impairment*).

Caveats to the IDEA (Individuals with Disabilities Education Act) Legislation

When a condition is being considered as a disabling condition under the IDEA umbrella, one has to consider the following caveats.

First of all, a medical or other diagnosis is *not* sufficient *by itself* to allow for special services or interventions. The condition must *adversely affect the student's* functioning, to the point that it jeopardizes full participation in the instructional day.

Secondly, services under IDEA are not intended to offer the *absolutely best* educational program possible for that student. Rather, it is intended to offer a program that is considered *reasonable* and *appropriate*. For example, a family and an 'outside' neuropsychologist (who has evaluated the family's tenth grader with PANS) might reasonably argue that, based on significant attentional problems and handwriting difficulties, the school district should cover the cost of a home/hospital tutor and an online program to teach their student Algebra. They may justify this need by saying that with such services, handwriting assignments will be minimal, and one to one attention will be assured. The school district, however, may counter that this is an unreasonable request. They instead may cite ways in which the student can still stay in the Algebra class with the regular Algebra teacher, with specific modifications and accommodations to help the student keep up.

Another important caveat to the IDEA legislation is that a child does not have to be failing in school to receive special education and related services. IDEA is designed to serve "any individual child with a disability who needs special education and related services, even if the child has not failed or been retained in a course or grade, and is advancing from grade to grade."[11]

Last but not least, it should be recognized that as of 2014, virtually *all of the states* in the US are, in effect, responsible for implementing services and educational programs under the federal guidelines specified by both IDEA and 504. (In the case of IDEA in particular, all states have accepted funding under its "spending clause" legislation, which makes them all subject to its statutes.) At the same time, some states interpret the provisions of IDEA more broadly than other states do (which in turn results in more services and help for the student). Especially in instances where the student may be relocating to another state, it is important to review these (possibly different) parameters with the departing IEP or 504 team, to assure that services and interventions will be continued in the student's new home state.

IDEA and the IEP

An essential element of IDEA is the provision for an **IEP** or **Individualized Educational Plan**. Typically, an IEP is thought of as a written, signed, and binding document that describes how the school district will meet the unique needs of a student with a disability. In reality, however, an IEP is actually a process that includes referrals, data gathering, assessments, collaboration across fields of expertise, student and parent input, implementation of agreed upon accommodations, interventions and services, and later, a review of its effectiveness. In other countries, such as Canada and the United Kingdom, an equivalent document is also called an *Individualized Educational Plan*.

Essential Differences between IDEA and Section 504: A Brief Comparison

The primary difference between **Section 504** and **IDEA** surrounds the design and implementation of an **IEP** and **Special Education**. Both offer procedural safeguards, such as avenues towards voicing grievances, but unlike Section 504, IDEA offers IEPs that are more specifically designed to address the student's unique learning abilities and disabilities, and that typically offer some sort of special education to address those needs. Moreover, because IDEA is more of an involved process, IDEA is often perceived as offering broader protections, accountability, timelines, and due process to students and their parents. In terms of procedural safeguards and protections, it may be helpful to note that, *IDEA is covered by the restraints and protections under Section 504, but not the other way around.* Again, it should be stressed that under both set of laws, however, there are avenues towards voicing noncompliance complaints.

Comparison Chart of Section 504 and IDEA

SECTION 504

- Civil Rights Legislation
- Reasonable accommodations for individuals with disabilities
- Federal Protections re: harassment of individuals in 'covered entities' because of their disabilities
- Requires schools to eliminate barriers that would prevent students from full participation in the general ed. Curriculum both on and off campus)
- Requires documented plan, but not an IEP
- Protects all participants in the program, including students, parents, and employees, from discrimination.

IDEA

- Federal Education Law
- Individualized Educational Plan, FAPE, LRE
- More procedural safeguards
- Typically viewed as offering better Expertise (more staff oversight) regarding the implementation of modifications and accommodations
- Special Education services range from a Least Restrictive Placement (i.e. in a regular education setting) to a Fully Restricted Placement (i.e. Residential School)
- Provides *supplemental* education and support

Parental Considerations towards an IEP vs. a 504

Some parents feel that if their child has an *IEP*, there is a better chance that their child will be more closely monitored by someone at the school who is knowledgeable about special education. They may also feel that this same person will be able to serve as a liaison with other staff members on what their child needs, and to make sure that an educational plan and services are appropriately being carried out. However, *technically*, the same could and should occur if the student has a 504 plan too.

Other parents may feel that *under a 504*, they maintain more control over what happens to their child's instruction. They may also fear that their child might not be exposed to the same curriculum as his peers, if he receives services that take him away from the "Regular Ed." classroom.

Implications of Legislation as it Relates to PANS in Public Schools

So, what can we glean from these laws, regarding the ways in which protections and support for students with PANS can be interpreted and expected?

1. **Access to a Free and Appropriate education.**

   Essentially, Section 504 prohibits discrimination against persons with a disability in any program receiving federal financial assistance, be it a public school or private school that receives any federal funding. This means that institutions are required to provide PANS-affected students with "reasonable and appropriate" access to learning and other school opportunities that *students who do not have PANS receive*.

2. **PANS as Limiting a Major Life Activity**.

   There are many symptoms associated with PANS that are clearly recognized to *limit one or more major life activities,* as defined by Section 504. Taken from the Office of Civil Rights own website,[12] this includes, for example, the ability to care for oneself, learn, sleep, read, concentrate, think, communicate, help, eat, or operate a bodily function.

3. **The Inclusion of Services Provided for Concomitant Conditions.**

   Regardless of whether students have a formal diagnosis of PANS yet or not, legislation specifically addresses many of its concomitant diagnoses. These include students with allergies and chemical sensitivities, mobility issues, Depression, Anxiety (or other mental health condition), "Attention Deficit Disorder (ADD)/Attention Deficit Hyperactivity Disorder (ADHD), and those who are medically fragile..."[13]

4. **The Recognition of Impairments Surrounding Bodily Functions.**

   Section 504 specifically addresses impairment of a "major life activity" surrounding *bodily functions,* where legislation clearly cites "**functions of the immune system**, ...digestive, bowel, bladder, neurological, brain, respiratory... and endocrine... functions."[14]

5. ***Limitations of a Life Activity* as Being Based on Comparisons with That Student's Age/Grade Cohort.**

   Critical to educational planning (especially when PANS symptoms are not yet diagnosed as PANS) "physical or mental impairment" is no longer limited to any *specific* disease or category of medical condition. A simple comparison with a student's *non-disabled age/grade peers* can suffice when determining whether an impairment is said to "substantially limit a major life activity" for the student.

6. **The Disallowance of *Mitigating Measures* as Grounds for Withholding Services.**

Section 504 in particular, acknowledges the aspect of 'mitigating measures.' Unless it is eyeglasses or contact lenses that are used to fully correct visual acuity, a school district *cannot rule out* the presence of a possible impairment on the basis that the individual has medications or treatment that might positively alter the condition.

An example of this would be if it were known that the student with PANS were taking prophylactic antibiotics, neuropsychiatric medications, or was scheduled to have an IVIG or Plasmapheresis treatment. Since 2009, Congress has specified that the "ameliorative effects of such mitigating measures must not be considered in determining if a person is an individual with a disability." [15] The aspect of mitigating measures is important to students with PANS, because it addresses and accommodates for its fluctuating nature (that comes with regression and healing over time).

7. **Expected Explorations (or Ruling out) of Even *Possible* Disabilities.**

Implicit in Section 504 and IDEA is the expectation that school districts will address the exploration of even *a possible* disability, through *Child Find* and other referrals. This, again, addresses the needs of those students with PANS symptomatology who may not have a clear definitive diagnosis yet. These guidelines also include conditions that are temporary in nature (6 months or less), episodic in nature, or in remission.

Moreover, in the US, in particular, school districts are mandated to consider findings of evaluations conducted by qualified examiners *who are not employed by the public agency* responsible for the education of the student in question. An **IEE**, or *Independent Educational Evaluation,* for example, should be considered for the assessment of any skill related to the student's educational needs *that are not addressed by those evaluators employed by the school district.* These may be obtained and paid for by the parents, but they may also be paid for the school district.[16] [17] Consistent with the mandates of US federal laws that provide an examination of all aspects of the suspected disability, referrals to outside evaluators can and should be made to rule out WHY behaviors and processing difficulties are happening. This information will, in turn, inform sound decision-making regarding HOW the educational program will appropriately serve this student. Pertinent to PANS symptoms then, this could possibly include the establishment of *parameters and the source* of changes in visual processing (as determined by a developmental or binocular vision clinic). It could also provide for the inclusion of an IHCP or school nursing plan, whereby a *qualified school nurse* develops a school nursing assessment and resulting school nursing plan to serve the student as he heals from the condition.[18]

Last, but not least, whereas school districts often limit assessments to that surrounding academic performance, US federal laws acknowledge that *educational performance* goes far beyond *academic performance to include* an evaluation in "all areas of suspected disability."[19] In other words, along with grades or other measures of *academic performance*, schools must examine the degree to which other factors, such as health, vision, hearing, social and emotional status, communication skills and motor skills may adversely affect the student's *non-academic* (as well as academic) performance too.[20]

8. **Access to Aids and Services (Regardless of Whether or not the Student is in Special Education).**

Under Section 504, students with PANS-related impairment have access to a number of aids and services that are available to ameliorate and support them in the educational setting. Specific examples include physical and occupational therapy services (the latter helpful for fine motor skill remediation, such as in handwriting); counseling, health services, speech and language therapy, transportation, etc. Moreover, one does not need to be receiving special education to obtain such aids and services.

9. **Bullying is Against the Law!**

Under both Section 504 and Title II of the Americans with Disabilities Act, students cannot be harassed in 'covered entities' because of their disabilities. School districts and postsecondary institutions are responsible to make sure that they are proactive in preventing bullying of students with behaviors that may be associated with PANS. Moreover, family members and teaching staff are legally protected as well.

10. **A Medical Diagnosis Alone Does Not Guarantee Services**

Students do not automatically qualify for Section 504 or IDEA (Special Education) based on a medical diagnosis alone. They do, however, if related symptomatology (such as anxiety, tics, enuresis, attentional difficulties, OCD symptoms, etc.) substantially limit the student's ability to perform a major life activity (i.e., school).

11. **Protections for Students for "Inappropriate Behaviors" Related to PANS.**

Section 504 and IDEA offer safeguards to disabled students regarding the improper removal from school for misconduct that is related to their disability. Before a district can implement a disciplinary action that constitutes a significant change in placement, a **"manifestation determination"** must take place. An evaluation must address whether or not the student's misconduct was caused by, or had a direct and substantial relationship to the students' disability, or was the direct result of the district's failure to implement the student's Section 504 plan. Moreover, a determination that the student knows the difference between right and wrong does not constitute an automatic determination that his misconduct was (or was not) a manifestation of his disability.[21]

If the team members determine that the disabled student's misconduct *is not* a manifestation of his or her disability, a district can discipline the student in the same manner that it disciplines non-disabled students for the same misconduct. However, if the student receives services under IDEA, special educational services may still be provided.

Additional Implications Regarding Services and Accommodations at Private Schools

A short review of related legislation clearly illustrates that even private schools can be responsible for providing certain services and accommodations to students with special needs. Although private schools are not required to offer special accommodations or services, they are required to do so if they receive any federal funding. Moreover, federal law provides funding to school districts for collaboration and consulting with private schools for students with disabilities who reside in those school districts. An additional consideration is that federal law *does not prohibit* services to take place at the private school (on the premise that *it is* a private school). This signals that the Student Study Team (which of course includes the parent) has some latitude in determining whether services will provided at the private school, and if so, what types of services will be provided.[22]

Moreover, many states require that school districts, upon request by the school, are obligated to provide services to students attending private school with health and welfare services, to that equivalent to those provided students in public schools. In the state of New York, for example, such services include, but are not limited to, "all of the services performed by a physician, dentist, dental hygienist, school nurse, school psychologist, school social worker and speech language pathologist. The services also may include dental prophylaxis; vision, hearing and scoliosis screening tests; recording health histories; physical examinations and in-school immunizations; maintaining cumulative health records; and administering emergency care programs for ill or injured students."[23] Whereas some state codes require that these services must be provided by the school district in which the nonpublic school is located, others specify that they be provided by school district *where the student resides*.

Private schools also open themselves up to scrutiny and legal action if they *advertise* that they accept and provide educational accommodations and services that have been previously documented by a recognized diagnostician, and then do not deliver on these promises. In general, however, it is acknowledged that, unless a private school is contracted by the public school district specifically to serve that student, or, if they receive federal funding of any kind, that any modifications or accommodations, testing, or special education will not be assured, guaranteed, or expected.

Implications of Legislation in Post-Secondary Education

For the most part, modifications, accommodations, and other services pertaining to postsecondary students are provided solely under the framework of Section 504, in that at this level of education, the student is least likely to need, or receive, special education *per se*. Moreover, most secondary (college, university, or other adult technical school) institutions are not designed for, nor do they receive funding for, the delivery of special education and other services (such as speech therapy) that the more comprehensive IDEA offers.

Under US law, at the elementary and secondary educational level, students with disabling conditions are entitled to a free and appropriate education, regardless of their level of skills or level of disabilities. At the postsecondary level, however, a student with a disability must also meet the academic and technical standards requisite for acceptance at that institution's educational program or activity. Moreover, whereas it is incumbent on the postsecondary institution to provide appropriate academic adjustments, auxiliary aids, and services to allow for *equal opportunity* to all students, they are not required to provide aids, services or adjustments that would result in a fundamental alteration of their programs or impose an "*undue burden*" on that institution.

At the college level, postsecondary institutions in the US adhere to guidelines set forth by state and federal legislation, such as Section 504. Under these parameters, a student *can* receive services and accommodations if she or he has a documented learning disability, medical condition, or psychological condition that warrants accommodations or modifications. Moreover, assistance is provided, regardless of what the student's former grades were, or history of being able to pass a grade level or standard has been. The student is generally entitled to receive accommodations, even if she has entered the college with a high grade point average, with no history of failed classes, etc.

A Timely Shift in Educational Paradigms- and Just in the Nick of Time

There have always been kind, creative, and thoughtful teachers, who, even without a legal mandate to do so, would informally and effectively address the needs of their 'atypical' learners to keep them on the educational track. This can certainly be said of many hard-working teachers today as well. However, it would only be natural to expect variations in the delivery of such accommodations, as so much would depend on the expertise, interest, time, and resources of the particular teacher and school. In looking at the educational codes of one's state, province, and nation, however, one can, at the very least, begin to sense *what would be within the expected parameters* for obtaining educational help and services, should they be needed. Often, parents and teachers are surprised to discover that, in fact, there is far more latitude in the depth and breadth of available help, than previously assumed.

In the last ten years, in the US especially, both legislation and curriculum have evolved to the point that, if implemented in the ways intended, real hope is offered to all students with special needs, including those students with such conditions as PANS. For example, Inherent in the legislation is the acknowledgement that services, special education, or both, are appropriate and reasonable for those with disabling conditions that may or may not be permanent. Legislation also acknowledges *variations* in cognitive ability, achievement, fluency rates, etc. This is important to consider, as PANS symptoms wax and wane. Perhaps most importantly, however,-for all concerned, is the recognition that in this case, the *illness is the source of fluctuations in achievement - and not the student's misbehavior, laziness, or lack of intellect per se.*

Of course, students maintain an important role in advancing their academic progress too, by being active participants in their own education (along with their medical recovery) as much as possible. Such participation includes continued participation in academic learning, as well as providing thoughtful feedback to providers on the efficacy of treatment, taking medications, and participating in prescribed therapies.

Curriculum and Pedagogy as Mirroring Legislation

This legislation also has evolved at a time when curriculum, surrounding both 'regular education' and the education of learners with special needs, has progressed too. No longer is it even marginally acceptable, to "dumb down" the curriculum for those sidelined in resource or special education programs to just "get them through school." At the same time, no longer should it be acceptable for those struggling in mainstreamed classes (think classes where most of the "neurotypical" students go) without the support they need to receive the curriculum of their peers.

In this way, **The Universal Design for Learning (UDL)** strives to meet the needs of all students (and whether they qualify for an IEP or 504, or not). As many US states have begun to implement the **Common Core Curriculum** in their schools, many have also looked to the fundamentals of the UDL to effectively reach all of their students with learning differences and special needs. In sum, the principles of UDL focus on the following:

- **Equal opportunities** to learn for all students.
- **Flexible approaches** that can be customized and adjusted for individual needs.
- **Multiple Means of Engagement** in the Learning Environment (the "why" of learning) -recruiting interest, sustaining effort and persistence; self-regulation.
- **Multiple Means of Representation** in the Learning Environment (the "what" of learning) –Perception, language, expressions, and symbols; comprehension.
- **Multiple Means of Action and Expression** in the Learning Environment (the "how" of learning) – physical action, expression and communication, executive function.[24]

An example of a lesson that is drawn from the principles listed above is provided in a later section. Our intent in citing UDL now, is simply to illustrate how progress in teaching philosophy has dovetailed legislation in its twin efforts to serve *all students*. This is undoubtedly an important change in pedagogical paradigms, especially considering the limitless array of intrapersonal and interpersonal strengths, challenges, and variations thereof, within our students with PANS.

In this section, we have looked at one nation's legislative backdrop that defines the parameters and expectations for educating its citizens with special needs. In Section V, we will move on to the specifics of obtaining actual services. What are the general processes that take place in this regard? What can one reasonably expect to occur at educational planning meetings? And, what avenues are available for parents and teachers to take when there are different views regarding what an 'appropriate' educational plan is? Section V will familiarize the reader with the *What's*, *Who's*, *When's* and *How's* of these educational processes, in order to provide a better understanding of the ways in which students can obtain the help they need.

Notes

[1] Section 504, Rehabilitation Act of 1973. (29 U.S.C. § 701)
[2] 34 CFR 104.
[3]29 CFR 1630.2
[4] 34 CFR 104
[5] 34 CFR 104.37
[6] Certainly, there is significant variation in the rights and access of students both in the US and worldwide to obtain a free and appropriate education. At the same time, unlike the United States, other countries may consider such education-related services (such as speech therapy or counseling) to be outside of the domain of Education, and may already provide them under their nation's health policy coverage.
[7] (76 FR 16977 federalregister.gov. 2011).
[8] Education for All Handicapped Children Act, 1975. Also see http://www.gpo.gov/fdsys/pkg/STATUTE-89/pdf/STATUTE-89-Pg 773.pdf.
[9] (IDEA Regulations: Part 300/A/300.8)
[10] (Taken from Federal Regulations: Part 300 / A / 300.8 / c / 9).
[11] Sec. 300.101 Free appropriate public education (FAPE). - IDEA
[12] http://www2.ed.gov/about/offices/list/ocr/504faq.html
[13] 29 Code of Federal Regulations1630.2) (29 CFR 1630.2.
[14] ibid.
[15] As cited in http://www2.ed.gov/about/offices/list/ocr/504faq.html.
[16] Taken from IDEA Regulations: Part 300 / E / 300.502 as cited in http://idea.ed.gov/explore/view/p/,root,regs,300,E,300%252E502.
[17] Sometimes the parent disagrees with an assessment that a district has done. When this occurs, the parent can request an IEE at public expense. At this point, the school district must then either fund the IEE or initiate due process to defend their evaluation. Moreover, the district is also allowed to put some parameters on the IEE in terms of qualifications of the potential assessor, etc., and the parent would have to make a case for any assessor who falls outside of the parameters.
[18] For many students affected by PANS, the inclusion of Independent educational evaluations (IEE'S) will be pivotal in the development of appropriate education plans that will accurately address their educational needs. For this reason, the following information regarding federal mandates is included here. Specifically, Sec. 300.502, which addresses Independent educational evaluations, reads as follows:
"(a) General.
(1) The parents of a child with a disability have the right under this part to obtain an independent educational evaluation of the child, subject to paragraphs (b) through (e) of this section.
(2) Each public agency must provide to parents, upon request for an independent educational evaluation, information about where an independent educational evaluation may be obtained, and the agency criteria applicable for independent educational evaluations as set forth in paragraph (e) of this section.
(3) For the purposes of this subpart--
(i) Independent educational evaluation means an evaluation conducted by a qualified examiner who is not employed by the public agency responsible for the education of the child in question; and
(ii) Public expense means that the public agency either pays for the full cost of the evaluation or ensures that the evaluation is otherwise provided at no cost to the parent, consistent with Sec. 300.103.
(b) Parent right to evaluation at public expense.
(1) A parent has the right to an independent educational evaluation at public expense if the parent disagrees with an evaluation obtained by the public agency, subject to the conditions in paragraphs (b)(2) through (4) of this section.
(2) If a parent requests an independent educational evaluation at public expense, the public agency must, without unnecessary delay, either--
(i) File a due process complaint to request a hearing to show that its evaluation is appropriate; or
(ii) Ensure that an independent educational evaluation is provided at public expense, unless the agency demonstrates in a hearing pursuant to Sec. Sec. 300.507 through 300.513 that the evaluation obtained by the parent did not meet agency criteria.
(3) If the public agency files a due process complaint notice to request a hearing and the final decision is that the agency's evaluation is appropriate, the parent still has the right to an independent educational evaluation, but not at public expense.
(4) If a parent requests an independent educational evaluation, the public agency may ask for the parent's reason why he or she objects to the public evaluation. However, the public agency may not require the parent to provide an explanation and may not unreasonably delay either providing the independent educational evaluation at public expense or filing a due process complaint to request a due process hearing to defend the public evaluation.
(5) A parent is entitled to only one independent educational evaluation at public expense each time the public agency conducts an evaluation with which the parent disagrees.
(c) Parent-initiated evaluations. If the parent obtains an independent educational evaluation at public expense or shares with the public agency an evaluation obtained at private expense, the results of the evaluation--
(1) Must be considered by the public agency, if it meets agency criteria, in any decision made with respect to the provision of FAPE to the child; and
(2) May be presented by any party as evidence at a hearing on a due process complaint under subpart E of this part regarding that child.
(d) Requests for evaluations by hearing officers. If a hearing officer requests an independent educational evaluation as part of a hearing on a due process complaint, the cost of the evaluation must be at public expense.

(e) Agency criteria.
(1) If an independent educational evaluation is at public expense, the criteria under which the evaluation is obtained, including the location of the evaluation and the qualifications of the examiner, must be the same as the criteria that the public agency uses when it initiates an evaluation, to the extent those criteria are consistent with the parent's right to an independent educational evaluation.
(2) Except for the criteria described in paragraph (e)(1) of this section, a public agency may not impose conditions or timelines related to obtaining an independent educational evaluation at public expense."
(Authority: 20 U.S.C. 1415(b)(1) and (d)(2)(A)) From: http://idea.ed.gov/explore/view/p/,root,regs,300,E,300%252E502
[19][20 U.S.C. Sec. 14(b)(3)(B)].
[20] [34 C.F.R. Sec. 300.304(c)(4)].
[21] In addition, a district cannot make a categorical determination that misconduct is or is not a manifestation of a disability based on a student's IDEA eligibility label.
[22] In these situations, students may have two sets of "Student Study Teams," one at the student's private school, and one with the student's home (public) school district.
[23] From the New York State Education Law 912. Taken from: *http://www.p12.nysed.gov/nonpub/handbookonservices/healthservices.html.*
[24] CAST, 2014. (Also see http://www.cast.org/our-work/about-udl.html#.VW-H1s9VhHw).

Section V

EDUCATIONAL MEETINGS AND PROCESSES TO PLAN AND ESTABLISH SERVICES AND INTERVENTIONS

The nature of obtaining special education or other educational accommodations and services in the United States is fairly prescribed, in that there are a number of federal and state laws that cover these services, primarily in public schools.

Most students with PANS will need some kind of educational accommodations or supports as they heal from this condition. That said, *not each and every student with PANS may need to go down this route of formalized plans and agreements.* In certain instances, the parent, in collaboration with medical and other providers and teaching staff, may choose to simply address symptomatology, informally as needed. The decision to proceed will absolutely depend upon a number of factors, including the severity and duration of the symptoms, the age, grade, and degree of regression of the child, and of course, the nature of the student's educational environment. The decision to proceed with more formalized planning and agreements will, however, assure that even in the event of a quick recovery and return to full academic function, that there is documented and binding confirmation by all parties on how that student's needs *have been*, and will *continue to be* addressed, especially in cases where a relapse may occur.

In the US, there are three primary avenues of service to consider when pursuing interventions and support for students with PANS. Due to the strong medical component of this potentially disabling condition, however, it is urged that a School Nurse be requested to be an integral part of the student study team, however one wishes to proceed. Depending upon the student, he may have an Individualized Health Care Plan or **IHCP**[1] (that primarily ensures interventions surrounding medical needs), a **504**, where it is acknowledged that the medical condition constitutes a disabling condition that warrants services, and/or an Individualized Educational Plan (**IEP**) (that typically requires some type of special education).[2]

Even if it is deemed that the student's health status *does not* require special education or a 504 plan, the family and school should still consider having an IHCP, especially if related symptomatology is suspected of affecting the student's school day. In general, components of a good IHCP also serve as an integral part of a 504 or an IEP as well.

General Steps in Obtaining Help under an Individualized Health Care Plan (IHCP)

1. The Student is Referred

Similar to those processes under a 504 or IDEA, referrals for an IHCP are usually made by the parent or guardian; however a referral can also be submitted by the teacher, support staff, medical provider, or others, if there is a perceived concern about the student's health and/or well-being. Written documentation should basically describe the reasons why the person is making the referral, and include the name, age, grade, and name of current teacher if in K-8. Moreover, it would typically include a request for a meeting with school officials to discuss the development of an IHCP.

2. Information is Gathered by the School

With an illness as broad reaching as PANS, an IHCP will provide for a School or District Nurse (or designee) to collect information regarding the illness's effects on the pupil. Here, the focus should not only include exchanges of documentation, but information gleaned from one-on-one interviews.

A scheduled, unrushed time to talk- with the people who are most knowledgeable and involved with the student's medical care and education- will yield a wealth of information regarding potential needs, services, and support. In this way, along with talks with the teacher(s) and other providers, a home visit, if it is amenable to the parent, not only serves to provide critical information, but just as importantly, serves to strengthen bonds of trust and collaboration among the school, home, and medical community during this time of crisis. (Although the following information is presented in the *format of **who** is being interviewed*, generally the timing of these interviews will overlap.)

I. Information is Gathered from the Parent or Guardian

A.) Health and Developmental History and Medical Information

These conversations will yield important information regarding the student's past and present health history. At a minimum, the nurse would conduct a health history that would include the following information specific to PANS:

- The date of diagnosis, and the establishment of where the child is at in the disease/treatment process.
- Perceived factors that could be affecting the student's regression or resilience.
- Any concomitant medical, psychiatric, or other types of diagnoses.
- The names and contact information of medical providers and others whom the interviewee might feel would be insightful sources.
- Specific health needs related to learning and participating in the school environment.[3]
- Current Level of self-care skills and needs.[4]
- Medications and related interventions in the past and in progress.
- Perceived effectiveness of treatment so far.

B.) A Review of Perceived Levels of Competencies Across Domains.

Conversations with the parent who sees the student at his best and worse will help establish how the following abilities, many of which are significantly affected in this student- have regressed, changed, or stayed the same since the onset of PANS. Of course, as the School Nurse discusses these aspects with the parent or guardian, she will be considering possible services or accommodations that could be of use at the school, and that she would recommend at the IHCP meeting.

In particular, the following topics would serve to provide the nurse or other evaluator with valuable information in which to help base a plan of future action. Such questions may focus on the student's current abilities to do the following:

- Demonstrate age appropriate self-care and daily living skills surrounding grooming, transportation, eating, etc. How long is it taking for the student to carry out grooming activities, such as bathing, dressing, and tooth brushing? Does the student experience upset, anxiety, or sensory overload in cars? (Are adjustments in attendance required?)
- Adapt to transitions and stresses common to the educational, home, and other environments, including and/or involving decision making, attendance, scheduling, and interactions with others. (Is a late-slip needed to be on file? Can the treating physician write a note to the effect that attendance in the morning is illness related?)
- Follow, understand, and remember written, oral, and visual information (and combinations of the three).
- Sustain focused attention for longer than 10 minutes (including activities that require listening, fine motor, and gross motor skills).
- Communicate effectively with others, and interact and behave in ways that are age-appropriate.

- Maintain social relationships. In what ways has his or her social life changed or stayed the same? How many times per month is the student invited to peers' homes, and what friends come to his home? Are friendships sought out?
- Complete chores, educational routines (i.e. homework), and other tasks of daily living in a timely manner.
- And, of course, the parents' views on their child's ability to acquire, and demonstrate knowledge (indicating the degree to which the student may need additional assistance, direction, and time to learn and to participate in an academic and other activities, such as in clubs, extracurricular activities, religious instruction, etc.).

C.) Areas Specific to the Student's Participation in School

As part of their health work-up, the school nurse or designee should consider some of the following activities that happen at home too, as they may directly affect the child's participation in school. Again, consider how these aspects have changed or stayed the same pre- and post-diagnosis and/or treatment.

- How many hours is the child actually sleeping each night? Sleep disturbances include night terrors, getting up to go to the bathroom, lying in bed awake, restless leg syndrome, etc.
- How has the child's diet and eating changed? Has the parent noted that certain foods are suddenly not tolerated any longer by the child? Have allergies, gluten or other sensitivities been noted by the parent or medical provider?
- How coordinated is the child in handling food? Is the child a messy eater? If so, is she or he aware of being messy? Does the child clean self and eating area afterwards?
- Have there been changes surrounding the sensory systems? Such areas would include any noted changes in functioning and any hyper/hypo sensitivities. In addition to addressing and monitoring status of hearing levels and visual acuity, consider other aspects of these sensory states on behavior and function, such as sensitivities to certain sounds or lights. (Should tennis balls on chair legs be considered?) Is he particularly sensitive to certain lights (halogen, florescent) or at certain times of the day? (Would curtains, a hat, or tinted sunglasses help?)[56]
- Have there been any changes in mood, parameters of mental health diagnoses, energy, stamina, affect, agitation, and unintended physical movements and utterances?
- What is the effectiveness of (and any observed side effects of) medications? These include those medications prescribed for ADHD, anxiety or mood, or other disorders. (It's important to keep in mind that some parents may not associate certain behaviors or conditions as being potential side effects of medications, especially in children.)
- How is this condition affecting the rest of family? Is the parent concerned over the child's safety, or the safety of those around him? (If so, how will the school apply federal safeguards and protections to assure that any behaviors secondary to the diagnosis of PANS will not result in inappropriate disciplinary techniques by the staff? A discussion with the parent on the disclosure of this illness to the police, should they be called, may also be warranted.)

Note: As the interviewer considers the parental responses, it is important to be aware of the differences in reports of perceived competence across the functional domains, *and by whom.*[7] What does any variance in interview responses (among home, school, and student responses) signal in terms of how PANS symptoms manifest in that particular student, and where?

II. Information is Gathered from Medical and Other Providers

If the student already has a PANS diagnosis, or if the student has already been seen by medical providers with concerns over their child's health, the parent or guardian should consider having the medical provider contact the school. This is facilitated by signing a **Consent for Release of Information Form**, which allows information to be exchanged among third parties (such as teachers with outside providers. Both the provider and the school will typically have forms allowing for this exchange. As a result, the nurse or designee will be able to contact the provider to secure the following:

- Confirm a diagnosis, obtain other information detailed in the Parent *Medical and Developmental History* Section above, and discuss all areas of concern related to the illness.
- Discuss any specialized needs that the student may need during the school day.
- Request that the medical providers' document other student needs, necessary supports, and services in writing.[8]

III. Information is Gathered from Teachers and the School Staff

During any discussions with the student's teachers, and when taking a cursory look over academic portfolios, report cards, and standardized measures (tests that compare the student's performance with same aged peers), the School Nurse should pay particular notice to the following:

- Evidence of fluctuating patterns of math grades, slower rates of task completion, worsening handwriting skills, skills of independent living, coordination, energy levels, attentiveness, and dips in social skills- especially as the warmer weather moves into the cold and flu season.
- The advancement or regression of his or her former academic skills and performance.
- Other perceived factors that could be affecting regression or resilience.
- Any perceived changes in his interactions with other students, in all environments of his school day (such as at recess, during breaks, and on field trips).

3. The IHCP Planning Meeting Takes Place

Information drawn from the above interviews and related documents will be used to provide the IHCP team with points to be covered at the IHCP. At most meetings, the following agenda items typically take place:

- Relevant paperwork and forms are handed out.
- Assessment data, gleaned from formal and informal measures and exchanges of verbal and written documents, is reviewed and discussed.
- Health problems/nursing diagnoses that summarize the student's health problems, and student's unique responses to PANS symptoms, are reviewed. Information may include the length of time the student has had the illness, the impact on school functioning, family variables related to the educational and medical care and support of this student, additional health conditions (such as allergies, etc.) and related medications.[9] [10]
- Goals Based on the above information, what are reasonable goals that can be put in place to address this student's needs as he recovers from PANS? (Goals may be short-term or long-term, but they must be measurable.)
- Interventions A nursing intervention is any treatment that is performed to reach a specific goal or desired outcome. These are listed along with the specialties of those responsible for their

implementation. Such specialists might include an *Occupational Therapist*, an *Adaptive Physical Education* teacher, etc.

- Expected student outcomes. Given the student's symptoms, what is expected to be accomplished *for*, or *by* the student, given the interventions (actions) that have been outlined? The outcomes must be *measurable* and related to the health problems/nursing diagnoses and goals.[11]
- The need for assistance is confirmed, and the details of the IHCP Plan is finalized, to include the following information:
  - What specifically will be provided?
  - Who will provide it?
  - When or how often will it be provided?
  - Where will it be provided?
  - When will it begin? When will it terminate?
  - How and how will it be monitored?
  - Who does the parent go to if questions arise? Who does the student go to if questions arise?
- The approval of the plan is signed to endorse, or not to endorse all *or parts* of the plan. If a participant does not approve of the plan, he or she does not have to sign it.

4. The IHCP Plan is Implemented

If team members feel confident that they have all of the information they need to develop an IHCP plan, the plan should be implemented.

The teacher and other designated staff and team members are expected to follow the strategies and procedures agreed to in the plan, and to participate in the review process. Teachers and other school staff listed on the IHCP plan are legally responsible to implement the designated accommodations/strategies/ services. Parents may also have a role in the implementation of some of the strategies.

- Teachers and other support staff should maintain records to document how they have attempted to implement the plan, and the effectiveness of the plan. These can include notations in grade books or files, and copies of submitted student work that has been adjusted or modified. This should also include pertinent communications with parents and other providers.

5. The Plan is Evaluated and Reviewed

- The goals and outcomes of the IHCP should be periodically reviewed, to also include the efficacy of interventions, and actual versus predicted outcomes.[12]
- Evaluations also should occur when the student's health status changes significantly or when the medical provider changes the student's prescribed treatment or medications.
- The IHCP should be reviewed at the beginning of every school year, at a minimum.
- Future meetings continue until an agreed upon IHCP plan takes place, or until an IHCP plan is no longer needed.[13]

General Steps in Obtaining Help under Section 504 and IDEA

Technically, the implementation of an IHCP may precede other supports and interventions provided under a **Section 504,** or it may not. Similarly, in the case of obtaining services under 504, many students with a medical condition (such as PANS) will be eligible to obtain accommodations, modifications, and other services *without* an Individualized Educational Plan (**IEP**) under the Federal legislation of the Individuals with Disabilities Education Act

(IDEA). It needs to be recognized only that the medical condition (PANS) *substantially hinders the student's ability to participate in, and/or keep up with the regular education curriculum.*

Similar to the IHCP, the implementation of a 504 may come before the decision to obtain an IEP, or it may not, again depending on the student's level of debilitation, duration of symptoms, age and grade level. Schools will often initiate services and other support through the 504 process, even though there is recognition that the student may later need special education too.

Very generally speaking, the *older* a student is at the time of a PANS diagnosis and related exacerbations, the *less likely* he would receive services under IDEA (in terms of receiving special education), and the more likely he would receive services under 504 only.[14] (This, of course, assumes that the student did not have other disabling conditions, prior to PANS, which may have affected his participation in the classroom.)

General Steps in the 504 Process

The 504 process involves five general phases, some of which overlap: referral, meeting(s), the development of a plan, the implementation of the plan, and the review of the plan.

1. The Student is Referred

Referrals can be made by the parent or guardian, the teacher, support staff, medical provider, or even a caring and observant relative or concerned custodian.

Child Find is a system included under both IDEA and 504 legislation, whereby public schools are charged to find children- whether they are attending public school or not- *who may be at risk of having a disability* that would make them eligible for services.[15]

For example, perhaps a teacher or playground supervisor notices that a previously engaged and athletic third grader is now spitting repeatedly on the tarmac at recess, and increasingly stays by himself as peers increasingly shun him when he attempts 'Wall ball' or other group games. Most of the time, the observer would probably notify the student's classroom teacher or principal regarding these changes. However, it would certainly be within the scope of Section 504 for the observer to make a formal referral for 504, as clearly, the student's behaviors suggest that a *"major life activity"* is likely being impaired.

Most of the time, however, it is usually the parent who makes the initial referral. This process can be initiated by a phone call or verbal discussion with school staff (usually the principal, the head of Special Education, or sometimes the school superintendent). *However, even if the initial referral is verbal, it is always best for the referral source to submit **written proof** of the verbal exchange.* This serves to establish a time line and written documentation in which to draw upon later. Written documentation should basically describe the reasons why the person is making the referral, and include the following information:

- Name, age, grade, and name of current teacher or counselor.
- Symptomatology affecting *(or even **possibly** affecting)* school work (tics, anxiety, forgetfulness, lethargy, poor attentional skills, poor fine motor skills, low energy, frequency of doctor's appointments, etc.).
- Examples of *known changes* regarding the student's ability to function or *fully* participate (in the classroom, in collaborative work groups with peers, on the playground, in PE, on field trips, etc.).
- Documentation of work samples or test scores that a parent or teacher has collected, and/or documentation from a medical provider citing the diagnosis and related areas of concern. (If the referral source chooses, he or she can hold on to these documents until the meeting.)
- In addition, the letter can request that certain people be invited to the planning meeting, such as the school nurse, speech therapist or others.

Typically, it will be the Case Manager or the 504 Coordinator who will telephone the parent or guardian to set up a time to meet, and also mail to them a notice specifying the agreed upon time and place of the meeting. Even though there are no required time lines specified in 504, meetings are expected to be held within a reasonable amount of time of receipt of the referral so that concerns can be discussed and a plan can be implemented. For this reason, most school districts adopt the same time line as is provided in the IDEA regulations.

2. The 504 Meeting Takes Place

The 504 meeting is usually held at the school or school district office, at a time agreed upon by the major attendees. At a minimum, the initial meeting might consist of the parent, the teacher and/or other referral source that is knowledgeable about the student, and an administrator. Often, if the administrator cannot be there, he or she will assign an **Administrative Designee** in her place. Basically the *Designee* speaks for Administration or School District, in determining whether or not the plan will be feasible, legal, and appropriate.

In some situations, there may be only one 504 meeting necessary to discuss concerns and devise an educational plan. These include instances where it is clear that only one or two accommodations or modifications will be necessary to keep the student in the regular education setting. (One example might include having increased access to the use of the bathroom during instructional hours. Another example might include having temporary accommodations or modifications surrounding logistical issues related to doctors' appointment times that conflict with school hours.)

However, unless additional testing or discussion is not needed, a 504 meeting will be the first of several meetings needed to develop a reasonable plan that will help the student. The following represents typical agenda items at a 504 meeting:

- **Participants Are Introduced**: After participants arrive, the case manager or the administrator will introduce all of the participants to one another. *Typically, there will only be one or two other people (in addition to the parents and teacher) who will meet.* However, depending upon the perceived need and expectations, team members at this meeting or future meetings can include:
    - <u>Family members</u>
    - <u>Educational and other school staff</u> (such as teachers, school nurses, occupational therapists, speech and language therapists, adaptive PE teachers, school psychologists, Special Education directors, District Advisors, and administrators)
    - <u>Outside medical providers</u> and therapists, such as psychotherapists
    - <u>Paid and unpaid educational advocates</u>
    - <u>Family friends</u>
    - <u>Other persons</u> deemed appropriate to be there, including clergy, Scout Leaders, and coaches, etc.
    - <u>The student</u> (The presence and participation of the student at these meetings will be largely dependent upon his age and developmental level.)

- **Relevant Paperwork and Forms** are handed out, including information surrounding **Procedural Safeguards**. These are to basically inform parents and guardians of what their rights are surrounding access to educational services for their child. Typically, this paperwork also lists contact information of agencies that will help parents obtain additional help, or recourse, should the school not provide the perceived interventions that were expected or needed.

- **Concerns** of the referral source and other participants are elicited and noted, along with written comments from those unable to attend. This includes positive feedback too, such as areas of strengths.

- Documentation is reviewed related to (in this case) either a PANS definitive diagnosis, a PANS (Rule-out) consideration for diagnosis, or symptomatology related to, or similar to PANS. Include related information from other providers.
- Relevant PANS symptomatology is detailed regarding how it affects full participation in the school day; (e.g. "Han's poor fine-motor skills limit the quality and quantity of his written work, etc.").

- **Regular education intervention strategies that have previously been used to assist the student, and their effectiveness, are reviewed**, as are any work samples, and documentation such as test scores, behavioral concerns and referrals, and anecdotal information to assist in the writing of the plan.

- **Specific accommodations, modifications or other services** are identified and discussed. (What will help the student maintain and further his abilities and progress best? For this student, would placement in the **least restrictive environment** be in a regular education classroom?)
  - Differing views are expressed and alternatives are suggested if there are questions or disagreements surrounding what is being said or recommended.
  - An **Assessment Plan** may emerge from this meeting if the team recognizes that additional testing will be appropriate. Alternatively, assessments may be offered and confirmed at this meeting, as well.

- **The need for accommodations, modifications, or other assistance is confirmed, and the details of the 504 Plan is finalized** to include the following information:
  - What specifically will be provided?
  - Who will provide it?
  - When or how often will it be provided?
  - Where will it be provided?
  - When will it begin?
  - When will it terminate?
  - How will it be monitored?
  - Who will be monitoring these services etc.?
  - Who does the parent go to if questions arise?
  - Who does the student go to if questions arise?

- **An appropriate review date is set**, in which parties meet and review the effectiveness of the 504 implementations.

- **The signature page is signed, whereby participants indicate *attendance* at the meeting**.

- **The approval of the plan is signed to endorse, or not to endorse all *or parts* of the plan.** If a participant does not approve of the plan, he or she does not have to sign it.

3. The 504 Plan is Implemented

If team members feel confident that they have all of the information they need to develop a 504 plan, the plan should be implemented. The teacher(s) and other designated staff and team members are expected to follow the strategies and procedures agreed to in the plan, and to participate in the review process. Moreover, those staff members listed on the 504 plan are legally responsible to implement the designated accommodations/strategies/services. Parents may also have a role in the implementation of some of the strategies.

- Teachers and other support staff should maintain records to document how they have attempted to implement the plan, and the effectiveness of the plan. These can include notations in grade books or files, and copies of submitted student work that has been adjusted or modified. This should also include pertinent communications with parents and other providers.
- Similarly, parents and guardians should also try to keep records of student work, and school- to-home verbal and written exchanges. This should include the parental observations of homework loads and completion of work pre- and post 504 implementation, student comments regarding school work and tests, staff feedback, and parental observation of student lethargy, mood, attentional skills, attitudes, and degree of school participation, post-504 implementation.
- If the teacher or staff member is concerned that the plan isn't working for the student, he should ask for the assistance of special education staff and other appropriate support staff (such as school counselors, nurses, or psychologists, etc.) The teacher or staff member should keep a written notation of when and who was asked to help in this regard.
  - *If the plan isn't working because accommodations or services are not taking place as agreed upon in the plan* (either because of logistical issues or other issues) this should be documented in writing as well, and referred to either the administrator or principal. This person is ultimately charged to address the non-compliance at the school level before moving on to the school district, mediation, or The Office of Civil Rights.
  - *If a parent or any other team member believes that the 504 plan is not working because it is not enough,* or *should be changed,* she should request a meeting (in writing) to the principal, with copies to team participants to discuss the limitations of the plan and to potentially adjust it accordingly. (The request to meet may not be necessary if there is already a planned review date listed on the 504 document already, and that will happen in a timely manner.)

4. The Effectiveness of the 504 Plan is Reviewed

- If at the meeting, the team reviews the effectiveness of the plan, and feels *that it is sufficient,* they may decide that no further meetings are necessary. In this case:
  - *The team continues to implement the plan as written, and unless concerns surface in the meantime-*
  - *A plan is made to reconvene each year, as long as adaptations, interventions and services for 504 are needed.*
- If, on the other hand, interventions or services are not going well or are *insufficient*, or there are issues or concerns that need further exploration (regarding a possible *impairment of a major life activity,* for example, (as noted in 504's definition), additional information or testing may be requested, and /or related aids, services or modification to regular education considered. Moreover, **Special Education** could also be considered. In this case, the team will proceed with asking for parental consent to initiate testing.
  - *The team decides on what additional types of evaluation(s),* if any, are necessary in order to assist the team with appropriate planning.
  - *The team then determines what types of modifications, accommodations or other services* should be provided in the interim.
  - *The team sets up a time to reconvene to discuss the results of testing.* Although under 504, there are no legal timelines associated with this review, school districts usually follow protocols under IDEA. In this case, this language states that the determination of eligibility as to *"whether a child*

is a child with a disability ... [shall be] ... within 60 days of receiving parental consent for the evaluation, or, if the State establishes a timeframe within which the evaluation must be conducted."[16]

- The team meets again to deliberate on the results of testing, to listen to those conducting the testing, and to discuss the results in terms of what it signals for accommodations and services. For example, a school psychologist might suggest the need for counseling once a week at school, based on the student's severe anxiety; the occupational therapist might urge that speech-to-text technology be used, based on their findings of weak fine motor skills; and the teacher might recommend that home/hospital instruction be considered, as the student's lethargy results in high rates of tardiness and absenteeism.
- Future meetings continue until an agreed upon 504 plan takes place, or until a 504 plan is no longer needed.

General Steps in the IDEA Special Education Process

Usually, the process of receiving services under Section 504 and IDEA will overlap, in that under IDEA, all of the procedures listed under Section 504 will be maintained and safeguarded. One significant difference between the two, is that under certain circumstances, testing or evaluations may not always be necessary under Section 504. With IDEA, there almost always is an evaluation period to determine services and eligibility.

1. The Student is Referred

- Even if parents speak to school staff in person or by telephone, a notification by letter, or at the very least, by email, is critical in that it will help establish time lines for follow-up meetings and services. These time lines are defined under the **procedural safeguards** related to IDEA. In this case, this language states that the determination of eligibility as to *"whether a child is a child with a disability ... [shall be] ... within 60 days of receiving parental consent for the evaluation, or, if the State establishes a time frame within which the evaluation must be conducted ..."* [17]
- The letter should include information regarding parental concerns re: PANS, and the effect it may have on their child's school performance (similar to that described under the 504 Section).

2. Planning and Placement Processes Are Initiated

Similar to the processes detailed under the IHCP and the 504, this course of action helps to determine the need for (and type) of evaluations. If needed, it also establishes interim help and support while more information is being obtained.

3. Evaluations Proceed

If the team decides on the need for more evaluations, these take place in efforts to guide decisions on obtaining special education and related services. Even without additional testing in place, however, the primary disabling condition of **Other Health Impairment (OHI)** should provide for *accommodations to take place in the interim* under Section 504 (i.e. *functions of the immune system*, etc.). This of course assumes that the student's health condition (PANS) also adversely affects his educational performance.[18]

4. Eligibility is Determined

The team uses the results of testing, which of course includes 'outside testing,' as well as input from treating physicians, behavioral health professionals, and others, to determine the disability and types of special education services needed/allowed under law. After this eligibility is determined, decisions are made regarding what goals are appropriate, what related, or other services, are necessary, and where any placements should take place.

Goals are designed to focus on those specific areas (such as in math or reading etc.), that one would want the student to achieve during the school year. Related services could include the provision for speech therapy, or the assignment of a one-to-one aide, or a note taker. Other services and interventions could include provisions surrounding teaching methodology (if, for example, the student's learning modality is limited to certain types of instruction). IEP teams also consider what is needed with regard to curricula (especially in comparison to what is taught at the student's grade level). Program modifications are discussed too (such as allowing the child to sit in an area of the room closer to the exit or bathroom). Provisions for transition planning and extracurricular activities, which can include sports and other after-school activities, are considered as well.[19] Programs and placement options are varied, based again on the specific needs of the student.

- Instruction in a regular education classroom, (and *continued* instruction in Advanced Placement Classes, Honors Classes, and classes for the Gifted and Talented when appropriate).
- Resource specialist services, where services can be provided in the regular education classroom or in a separate classroom for part of the day.
- Special classes that serve students with similar types of conditions, and more intensive needs.
- State special schools.
- Home or Hospital instruction for all or parts of the school day.
- Instruction in hospitals or institutions, such as medical facilities, state hospitals, and juvenile facilities.
- Placement in nonpublic non-sectarian schools when no appropriate public school placement is available.
- Residential placements, including non-medical care, and room and board when educationally appropriate, or when the only appropriate school is too far away from the student's home.
- Instruction using telecommunication.
- Itinerant instruction in classrooms or other settings, where specially designed instruction may occur.[20]
  - *Note:* The school district is obligated to consider the type of learning environment that will be *least restrictive* for the student. In instances then where a *more restrictive* placement is recommended, the IEP team must document reasons for such placements.

5. All or Parts of the Plan are (or are not) Agreed Upon

If the child is found eligible for services, team members sign their consent towards the agreement of all, or part, of the recommendations. For example, the parent may feel that some of the components *do* address their child's needs, but that others *do not*. They may also agree with the goals and objectives of the plan, but they may disagree with *the actual placement site,* or location, in which such services will be carried out. Similarly, the *school district* may feel that the recommendations of the proposed IEP (with which the parent doesn't agree with) *are* necessary. In either case, legislative procedural safeguards allow for **mediation** or **Due Process** procedures to help resolve these issues.[21] While these issues are pending, however, the student remains in his current classroom placement, unless the team agrees otherwise.

6. An Individualized Educational Plan (IEP) is Implemented

If the child is found eligible for services, special education and/or related services must be implemented within a given time from the initial date of referral (above).

7. The Effectiveness of the IEP is Reviewed

The effectiveness of the plan is reviewed, along with additional and comprehensive testing occurring at least every three years, and with annual meetings (or more if needed) expected to occur.

Student Study Team Planning and Assessment Considerations Specific to PANS:

Thinking of the Big Picture Going In

As parents, case managers, teachers, and administrators prepare to develop an effective educational plan tailored to this student's needs, they should be aware that PANS symptomatology presents a unique set of parameters that are highly variable. Symptomatologies vary not only from these students' previous levels of function and from their 'neurotypical' peers. They vary from many other students within the world of "*special education/ 504/IHCP*" needs. Therefore (and regardless of whether or not a student is being served under a 504 or an IEP process), the following considerations are warranted.

1. Collaboration with the Treating Physician/Medical Provider

Collaboration with the treating providers must be initiated as soon as possible, to determine the nature of the illness, and to learn how this condition would affect the child's work/ stamina at school.

2. Close Collaboration with the School Nurse

The school or district nurse is in the best position to collect and interpret health information to the team, and to serve as an appropriate liaison among the medical provider, the parent, and the school).

3. The Procurement of an Academic Portfolio of Work, and Results of Evaluations Previously Completed

It is especially important to contrast present academic performance with former performance, paying particular attention to what is demonstrated under the constraints of the illness.

4. Age of the Child

Very generally speaking, the younger the child, the more comprehensive testing needs to be, in terms of guiding treatment and providing other educational services (such as Speech Therapy and Occupational Therapy, etc). Again, generally, if the student has already met most of his age-appropriate milestones before diagnosis, there may less of a 'recessed level of foundational skills' to catch up on later. Therefore, although it is true that there certainly can be regression with newly diagnosed middle schoolers or high school students, a student's continued mastery in certain functional domains may signal the need for limited testing only, (such as that pertaining to handwriting ability, reading speed, test-taking abilities, etc.).

5. Stamina Levels for School and for Testing Sessions

Pay close attention to the student's present levels of attention, distractibility, and overall energy, which may affect the outcome of testing. It is important for the school to have feedback from the parent too, in this regard. Carefully determine the student's cognitive and/or physical stamina to complete long (or even short) batteries of tests.

Certainly, testing results may be compromised by the severity of the illness during the time of the assessments. At the same time, however, if the student is tested during a *waning* period (when symptoms are far less marked), results may illustrate abilities, but not the types of hindrances reflected during a *waxing* period.

6. How is Testing Going to Guide or Provide Services?

The question must be *"How would these test results initiate and inform a discussion of how my child can better keep up with the regular education curriculum- to the best of his/her ability?"*

7. The Inclusion of Outside Testing Results

Testing results often include evaluations elicited from "Outside" the school system. These can include Binocular vision evaluations, neuropsychological testing, ImPACT testing, etc. The results and recommendations from such *outside* testing can often "get the ball rolling," in terms of providing 504 accommodations, at the very least. Moreover, legislation acknowledges that districts can cover testing by an outside provider if it addresses the evaluation of a possibly disabling condition and it is recommended by the student study team IEP. This usually happens if there is no one deemed certified or competent to provide the specific assessment on the school staff (such as a developmental optometrist or an occupational therapist). (There are also certain provisions for the district to pay for an evaluation from an Outside provider, if the parents disagree with the results of the evaluation that is conducted by the school district.)

8. Little Likelihood of "Specific Learning Disability"

Many students with PANS- at this point in time anyway- will **not** qualify for special education services under "**Specific Learning Disability**."[22] If teams are looking to determine a *specific learning disability* (using a substantial discrepancy between ability and achievement), this may not always be apparent. This is often because their ability, or aptitude scores (drawn from their performance on tests of memory, verbal skills, and fluid reasoning, etc.) may not be that much higher than their (often strong) achievement scores (such as reading, writing, and math abilities, etc.). For many students with PANS, their achievement scores (heavily based on performance yielded from earlier pre-PANS learning ability and efforts will be "too high" to be considered "weak" enough to warrant the diagnosis.

9. Testing as a Transitional Glimpse

It must be acknowledged by all parties, including team members, family members, and, as much as possible the student himself, that testing results merely provide a *transitional glimpse* of abilities. It is important to recognize that dips in performance are associated with PANS, and can be expected. However, it is just as important to be mindful that the long-term trajectory of this illness is excellent. Taking this positive trajectory into account then, what provisions will there be for *follow-up testing,* as symptoms improve? And, if there are no provisions for future testing, what will be 'the narrative' surrounding the results of this current testing in the student's future? (In other words, will all parties, including the student, be clear in their understanding that those low scores were tied to PANS' symptoms, and NOT to the student's intrinsic aptitude, etc.?)

10. Emphasis on OHI as the Primary Disabling Condition

In most cases, the "learning disability" is symptomatic (and secondary) to PANS. Many will need services, and in the US, will qualify under the disabling condition of Other Health Impairment.

Areas of Testing Most Relevant to PANDAS/PANS

Let us review the *types* of testing that should be considered when determining the needs of students with PANS. As stated previously, PANS touches on many domains of function. Predictably then, these would correspond to a number of areas that could warrant examination. Listed below are the general areas that are typically looked at. In looking at the following list, one will quickly notice how many of the areas overlap. For example, fine motor skills and visual processing are both needed for handwriting, and for other types of eye hand coordination.

- Tenets explored in a School Nursing Evaluation (consistent with an Individualized Health Care Plan).
- Fine Motor/Visual Motor skills (to include handwriting ability, drawing and copying of images, etc.[23]
- Visual Processing (acuity, convergence, tracking, closure, speed, etc.)

- Auditory Processing/ Language Processing, involving receptive language (What are they understanding?) and expressive language (*What* are they, and *how* are they effectively communicating with others?)
- Memory Skills (Visual and Auditory- separately, together, and sustained.)
- Executive Functioning Skills (attention, planning, self-monitoring).
- Sensory Integration/Sensory Defensiveness (tactile, visual, auditory and olfactory). The team has to know how to recognize certain triggers that will result in sensory overwhelm for the child; the team then has to put a plan in place to mitigate triggers or help the child accordingly.
- Adapted PE/Gross Motor/Recreational. (Don't forget what is happening on the playground.)
- Functional Behavior Assessment (to include information about how the student is actually functioning across different domains (such as grooming, obtaining transportation, and self-help skills.
- Social/ Emotional Development. (Again, how do they demonstrate age and gender appropriate skills in their exchanges with others, and by their behaviors? How well do they 'self-regulate' their reactions when things are not going well, etc.?)
- Assistive Technology. (How could computer software etc. aid them academically? Do they need such technology that will "read" highlighted text on a computer screen, **"text to speech**" to help them keep up with reading, etc? And what programs and what type of instruction in the use of this technology would be appropriate?)
- Present Levels of Achievement in Reading, Writing, Math, Oral Language, and other subject matter skills consistent with grade level.
- Comparison of Present Academic Achievement Levels in reading, writing, mathematics, and other academic portfolio work, with past achievement.
- Assessment and Interviews That Will Yield Information on Transition Planning. (This includes going from different levels of education to higher levels, and especially includes transitioning from secondary school to college or other training facility, or employment.)
- Psychiatric, Medical, Optometric, Audiological, and Speech, Occupational, and Physical Therapy, as well as other fields of expertise, may be needed to appropriately evaluate this student's areas of concern. In these cases, outside referrals to conduct evaluations may be appropriate.[24]

Important Distinctions between Accommodations and Modifications

Both Section 504 and IDEA provide **accommodations** and **modifications** to eligible students. However, there are distinctions between the two.

Accommodations

Accommodations are generally adaptations to the ways in which learning is taught, and subject content is assessed or measured. Accommodations allow the student to demonstrate what he or she knows without fundamentally changing the target skill that's being taught in the classroom or measured in testing situations. For example, a student with attentional problems secondary to PANS might need to take a test in a separate 'distraction free' room to stay focused and complete his work. Generally, accommodations surround the use of *timing* of a task or a test (such as having extra time or allowing frequent breaks), and *setting* in which tasks will be completed (a 'distraction free' room instead of a classroom, or the use of study carrels etc.) Accommodations also address changes in *how* the material or knowledge will be demonstrated by student (written, oral, Braille, etc.?) and *how* it is presented or learned.

Modifications

When schools refer to modifications, they are usually referring to *adaptations* to instruction or to assessments. Typically modifications change or reduce the target skill in some way. For example, a student with PANS may spend two to three times as long as her peers to complete homework or tests, because of related anxiety or handwriting difficulties. The team might recommend modifications to assignments, and even tests, which require her to only complete *every other* item, or write shorter papers, or do alternate projects, etc. Another modification might be for the teacher to *substitute* a crossword puzzle assignment with an alternate assignment that wouldn't require a high level of eye hand coordination.

Curriculum modifications for this student might include being excused from particular projects, or learning different material while others in the class are doing something else. Still, another curriculum modification for the PANS student might be that he be graded or assessed with a different assessment standard than what the instructor is using with classmates. For example, whereas others in the class might be graded on the "proper use of adverbs" by how well they did on a *"written test worth 100 points at the end of the term,"* this student would be graded or evaluated on the "*percentage of instances"* that he *"correctly demonstrated the proper use of adverbs in essays that were submitted during the last two months of the grading term."*

Concerns are often voiced, and sometimes quite rightly, that modifications can sometimes "water down" the curriculum, and put into question the validity of the student's true command of material. However, with creative, thoughtful, and careful implementation and monitoring of such modifications, students' attainment of curriculum content can be assured. Moreover, modifications, when used appropriately, are considered to be an integral part of the delivery system of the **Universal Design for Learning (UDL),** which along with the **Common Core Standards** has been embraced by most state Departments of Education in the US.

Such alterations to student work or curriculum can not only be beneficial, but absolutely essential to students who are experiencing PANS exacerbations. For many students with PANS, a prime example of this surrounds the extraordinary demands of homework completion. As work continues to accumulate, and these students struggle harder and harder to keep up, they run the risk of falling further behind, both in their *past school work,* and in their *current school work*. Over time then, they will predictably miss more and more of the *foundational material* that the rest of the class has already mastered, and that is now used as a base for what is *now* being taught. What is worse, however, is that as these students fall further behind, they may also succumb to increased levels of stress, despair, and low self-esteem, as they experience 'success' becoming less and less within their reach.

The Important Role of the Case Manager, 504 Coordinator, or Designated Liaison

The pivotal role of the person, who in many cases, is responsible for assembling a school team, delegating responsibilities, and collaborating with others to produce an effective educational plan for the student, cannot be overestimated. This will be true, whether she has the support of legislative backing, or not.

In the US, for example, regardless of whether or not the student is receiving services under Section 504 or IDEA, every public school, and *every private school that receives any federal funding,* should have a designated 504 Coordinator. This person, for example, is responsible for monitoring and assuring that tenets and protections under 504 civil law are being carried out appropriately. It is very helpful, (though not required legally), that the 504 designee has a background in special education practices. It is *imperative* however, that the individual is practiced and knowledgeable regarding the delivery of services and current legislation, be she the case manager for *a 504,* or *Special Education/IDEA* process. It is also extremely helpful if the coordinator is *familiar with those individuals/specialists* who are involved in the delivery of services and special education in that school and school district. A good, experienced case manager or 504 Coordinator, unlike a novice, will be aware of *alternate routes* to get the student (and teacher) services and help that they need. She will also be aware of the internal politics, staff personalities and expertise, and specific budgetary constraints that collectively, have the potential to create (or alternatively, limit) a good educational outcome for this student.

Schools and school officials may certainly vary in their procedures, and willingness, to provide services to students with special needs. Even in uncertain and challenging environments though, a knowledgeable and skilled case manager can often be a better advocate for the student. She will be able to provide a more comprehensive discussion with all parties (teachers, administration, outside providers, etc.) regarding what *actually is possible* (or considered "reasonable and appropriate") under the related laws, and just as importantly, *what is not*. Moreover, parents and teaching staff need to feel confident that the person is able to work effectively, realistically, and fairly with all concerned on the student's behalf. Good communication skills with teachers and other staff, who may or may not understand (or accept) the use of modifications and accommodations in their classrooms, will be critical to the implementation of *any plan*, be it one under 504 or IDEA.

Teachers must also feel confident that *their* feedback, based on their opinion of the student's school work, test scores, and observations, is taken into account in planning and decision making. They must also feel confident that they will be supported with staff assistance, guidance, planning time, and technological equipment, if necessary, to effectively carry out accommodations and services. In this regard, and very realistically speaking, teachers *must trust* that the 504 Coordinator or Case Manager will not "dump" additional responsibilities at their feet, that will put them in a position that they either have no training or support to carry out effectively, or that will, in any way, modify the conditions of their employment contract.

For example, let's take the case of a student in the US who, because of his disabling condition, qualifies for having a designated school bus transport him home after school. In this particular instance, an administrator (who is at the meeting) is aware that the bus company cannot pick up the child until forty minutes after the regular instructional day, without the district being subjected to a significant increase in transportation costs. To avoid the additional strain on the transportation budget, the administrator may urge that the teacher use this forty minute period to allow for "*additional educational goals and objectives*" to take place. The parent enthusiastically responds that this would be a "wonderful way" for her child to get the extra help he needs. In this case, the 504 Coordinator or Case Manager would be looked upon to provide guidance and boundaries consistent with related laws pertaining to both the educational care of the student, *and* the employment protections and contracts of the staff. She would consider all of these parameters, *along* with the recognition of student need. She then might suggest that an alternate plan be put in place. For example, if she were aware that this instructional time would supersede the teacher's contracted instructional minutes, she might recommend that a para-professional be hired to work with the student instead.

Notes

[1] Depending upon where the student lives, this plan might also be referred to as an **IHP** (individualized Health Plan), **ICP** (Individualized Care Plan), or something else.

[2] For a deeper discussion regarding the educational planning for *post-secondary* students with PANS, see Section VI.

[3]From the State of Virginia Department of Education 12/2014 (retrieved July 2015). http://www.doe.virginia.gov/support/health_medical/specialized_health_care_procedures/appendix_a.pdf

[4] ibid.

[5] Also regarding vision, a Binocular vision examination is strongly urged, because regardless of their visual acuity, most will experience significant weaknesses in visual fluency (especially when paired with fine motor demands.

[6] Regarding visual processing impairments, rule out convergence insufficiency (where both eyes have difficulty teaming up to focus at different various distances efficiently).

[7] Feedback may differ considerably depending upon who one is talking with. Typically, the parents will assess lower functional levels of their child. This is partly because the student may put a tremendous amount of energy to 'self-censure' aspects of the illness when he is at school or in public. Parents may report that at home, there is more latitude and perceived safety by the student to be able to "fall apart." At the same time, however, it is recognized that, in fact, there is a "nesting nature" to one of the primary diagnoses related to PANS- Obsessive Compulsive Disorder. In this case, behaviors are triggered by activities that tend to take place at home, such as grooming, eating, and dressing.

[8] An example of the types of supports a provider might include is listed in the appendix.

[9] The NANDA-I Web site at http://www.nanda.org has developed a related listing of health problems that can be useful in this regard.)

[10]A nursing diagnosis also defines what the school nurse can contribute as an autonomous practitioner. (State of Virginia Department of Education).

[11]You may find the Nursing Outcomes Classification (NOC) can be helpful and are available online at http://www.nursing.uiowa.edu/cncce/nursing-outcomes-classification-overview).

[12] State of Virginia Department of Education.

[13] South Carolina Department of Education August 8, 2013 Mick Zais, Ph.D. State Superintendent of Education has an excellent review of necessary tenets in this regard.

[14] Candelaria Greene, J. F. (2015) Unpublished survey of family members, providers, and survivors of PANS regarding PANS and Education, collected as UC Berkeley Research Scholar, Berkeley, California (2013-2015).

[15] In procedural guidelines taken from the North Region SELPA Procedural Guidelines Handbook, it is stated that "Each school district shall actively and systematically seek out all individuals with exceptional needs, ages 0 through 21, including children not enrolled in public school programs and students who are migrant, homeless, or wards of the State, that reside in the district or are under the jurisdiction of the SELPA or county office. All districts should have adopted policies for notifying parents of their rights and for initiating a referral for assessment to identify individuals with exceptional needs. For students from birth to 3 years of age, school districts only have child find responsibilities for children with low incidence disabilities (deafness, blindness, and /or orthopedic impairments)". (North Region SELPA Procedural Guidelines Handbook, 2015)

[16] IDEA 2004 at 20 USC 1414(a)(1)(C)(i)(I)" (Taken from (Wrightslaw: Special Education Law, page 93).

[17] ibid.

[18] As explained further in Section IV under the discussion of OHI.

[19] Siegel, L. (2005) The Complete IEP Guide How to Advocate For Your Child. 4th Ed. p 10/9. Nolo Press, Berkeley. (Nolo Press offers this as an excellent guide in general for advocating for the child with special needs.)

[20] Samples of placements taken from *Information on IEP Process* 10/9.http://www.disabilityrightsca.org/pubs/504001Ch04.pdf.

[21] The IEP due process is protected under IDEA legislation, and provides parents with the right to resolve disputes with the school district. In mediation, the parent and a representative of the school district meet with a neutral third party, who then tries to help both parties reach a solution. The mediator has no authority, however, to impose a decision. They are paid by the government to help parties resolve disputes. If a decision can't be reached through mediation, or parties wish to request a due process hearing directly, written evidence and witnesses are presented before a hearing officer. Even then, if parties do not agree with the outcome of that hearing, they can appeal the decision all the way to state or federal court.

[22] 'Specific Learning Disability' is one of the disabling conditions used to determine eligibility for services and accommodations under IDEA.

[23] These types of testing are often provided by an Occupational Therapist or school psychologist.

[24] Depending upon where the student lives, these may be provided for within the school district or within the national or state health care provisions. These include MOA's (Memorandum of Understandings) with providers outside of the school district, per se.

Section VI

ACCOMMODATIONS, MODIFICATIONS, AND SUPPORT STRATEGIES

Translating Special Needs into Educational Practice: The 'Broken Leg' Paradigm

An easy way of thinking about a *'504'* and Special Education- and presenting it to those who may be reluctant to accept such measures- is to think of it in terms of the *'Broken Leg Paradigm.'* Let's say that a student has broken her leg while playing sports. *Of course* that student would need to use an elevator or ramp to get to classes. Similarly, if a student injured her dominant arm or hand, *of course* she would need to have someone take notes for her, or dictate test responses instead of writing responses down. In these instances, students do not need special education or remedial instruction. They can *learn* the material adequately enough; they just need some accommodations and modifications in their learning environment to better *access the information* and to *demonstrate their knowledge*.

Moreover, when it comes to serving students affected by PANS, the notion of the *Broken Leg Paradigm* goes even further than simple modifications and accommodations. This is because PANS takes a hit (albeit temporally) on a number of *cognitive processes* that are needed to progress academically. As a result, (and especially if the student has suffered from the illness for an extended period of time) she may need some sort of individualized or special instruction. Such ancillary instruction- in a resource class, or with an assigned instructor in special education or in another subject matter, will help safeguard this student's ability to maintain the skills she *does have* as she progresses through the curriculum. In this way, there will only be minimal, if any, 'lost ground' once her health fully returns.

Therefore, the justifications for providing a 504 **or** an IEP to a student with PANS are one and the same. PANS symptomatology, related to changes in mood, attention, academic fluency, and processing rates, (but also related to an increased need for bathroom breaks, an onset of tics, or hypersensitivity to lights and sound, etc...) will, *of course,* result in the need to implement services to help accommodate for such factors. The student should be assured that such accommodations and instruction are not giving her any unfair advantage. If anything, such measures are only helping to ensure that a *level playing field* is in place; one, where she can keep up with her peers in the most **appropriate** and **least restrictive** grade, curriculum, or class, as she heals from the condition.

Before one proceeds through the following pages, it bears repeating that, as there is no *one-size-fits-all* presentation for students who are stricken with PANS, there is also no *one-size-fits-all* educational plan for them either. The earlier and the more promptly these students are correctly diagnosed and treated, the less likely they will go on to suffer regression, dysfunction, and periodic waxing and waning of symptoms. Some students, in fact, may return to their 'baseline skills and abilities' immediately after completing treatment (and never regress again). Therefore, the reader should be aware that these pages represent a *range* of services, rather than a prescriptive for any and all diagnosed students.

Part 1: Supports to General Areas of Need

Health Supports and School Nursing Supports

- Involve the School Nurse, Parents, Teachers, and Staff
  In addition to the supports provided by an Individualized Health Care Plan (IHCP), Student Study Team members should be periodically and regularly kept apprised of updates on health and other related information that could affect student progress. Moreover, as part of the IHCP, an emergency plan should be considered. This would include sudden changes in health and behavior, and would also

include contact information, medications and allergies, procedural safeguards necessary for fieldtrips, etc.

- Modify Attendance Policy if Necessary
  Owing to changes in sleep, mood, and schedules surrounding health status and doctors' appointments, etc., a modification in attendance may be necessary. Along these lines, but within the parameters of keeping placement in the least restrictive environment, the team may also want to investigate the benefits of having a home/hospital tutor for part of the day and during periods of waxing symptoms.
- Establish Health Alert
  In addition to establishing staff awareness of any special needs that the student has regarding allergies, food sensitivities, and sensory triggers, they should also be made aware of protocols for informing the family if Strep or other contagious diseases are reported at school.
- Develop a PANS Awareness Program
  As per student or parent request and/or collaboration, a PANS awareness program may be offered within the school district, or sometimes even in the classroom (as again, per student comfort levels).
- Provide School Counseling, and Provide Links to Outside Providers When Appropriate.
  The school counselor can serve as a valuable liaison and resource for both the student and the family. In addition, her office may also serve as a refuge during periods of waxing symptoms. Remember that such services can also be extended to family members too, if it is integral to the educational support of the student.
- Provide Access to a Staff or Otherwise *"Safe"* Bathroom Throughout the Day (and Provide a Permanent "Bathroom," "Hall Pass," or other Type of Arrangement, as Long as it is Needed
  It is acknowledged that a noted symptom among these students is an increased need to void. However, the need to 'go to the bathroom' serves other purposes too. These include such varied reasons as the need to move, the need to find refuge where one can express tics without being looked upon (and judged) by others, and the need to take a mental break from classes that have become overwhelming, etc. Moreover, it should also be kept in mind that the student might want to use the bathroom *only* during class hours, to avoid potential negative interactions *(i.e., taunting or harassment)* with students who would regularly use the bathroom during recesses, etc. Whatever the reasons are, these students should not be questioned in this regard, but allowed to use the bathroom upon request.
- Arrange for Extra Personnel on School Field Trips
  This may be necessary for the administration of medications, or if it's known that assistance on long walks or on rugged terrain will be necessary. In some instances, these students may become tired and hot easily, and they may need to rest more than their peers. To the extent possible, the student should be able to participate in a variety of field trips, even if it is in a limited capacity. The key to successful participation is adequate planning and staffing.
- Provide Assignments and Alternative Educational Placements with Hospital/Home School When Necessary
  In instances where the student is at home or in a hospital, arrange for communications and assignments to be exchanged. Consider the use of interactive systems, such as Skype and the use of email, etc.
- Arrange for the Student to Leave Class Early to Get to the Next Class
  This student may need extra time to transition to the next class, due to symptoms of lethargy, problems with organization, or other factors associated with this illness. Preferential seating near an exit will allow the student to leave and enter classrooms with less disruption and attention.

- Provide Referrals to Therapeutic Supports and Other Specialty Providers (such as hearing and vision specialists), as needed
  Also, under law, such ancillary services can be provided by the school district, in cases where it is seen as pivotal to the educational support of the student.
- Consider Transportation Needs
  PANS sufferers are often sensitive to car and other types of travel. In these instances, attention must be made to both the *triggers* that can make trips to school (and to other affiliated trips) difficult, along with *modifications or implements* that can make trips bearable. For example, the student may be given preferential seating (near the front, where he can look straight ahead, thereby reducing an overwhelming sensation of vehicle movement). He may be provided with headphones that bar noise, a comforting toy or pet, or the use of an electronic game that can help make the trip more soothing. Such travel becomes especially critical to consider on trips of over ten or fifteen minutes, where there may be only one adult accompanying the student, and where that adult is also the driver. In this case, a transportation 'aide' may be necessary. If the IHCP/Student Study Team is considering the services of "outside agencies,"[1] such as therapists, etc., they must rule out and/or address the potential hardship of transportation *on both the student and the parent.* Without taking this aspect of educational planning into account, such travel can become difficult, and sometimes dangerous, rendering any rationale for the journey (i.e., therapy) of uncertain value.
- Provide Awareness of how Medications, Specific Foods, and other Environmental Agents Can Affect Behavior
  As with students *not* affected by PANS, foods and medications can impact behavior and learning in a number of ways. The School Nurse, teacher, and parents should be kept abreast of both positive and negative changes observed as a result of modifications in medications, supplements, foods, and other potential 'triggering' agents. Some students may have specific needs that emerge when they change medication regimes. In these instances, students may require periods of rest, increased intakes of water or snacks, or a decreased work load. Some may even require a decrease or increase in physical activity.
  Staff must adhere to guidelines regarding dietary restrictions (including potential gluten intolerances, food sensitivities, etc.), as intake of certain foods or food additives in affected children can result in significant cognitive and behavioral changes, along with changes in health.[2] (Often parents are willing to bring in allergen-free foods for parties or events if they know in advance of the function.)
- Facilitate Assistance For Social Involvement
  It is important to recognize that a part of the school experience is the social aspect. Remember that participation in extracurricular activities is safeguarded under law. The team should consider how that student can be kept abreast of what is going on at school, and how he can still maintain inclusion in the social aspects of the school program (such as participation in clubs, graduations, dances, sports, or other events). Moreover, the team must assure that to the extent possible, relationships cultivated within safe and positive social groups are either maintained or facilitated. These can include having lunch with a favored teacher or staff member in their classroom, where students can feel safe and supported. Moreover, the nature of this student's social interactions should be monitored, as changes in their quality and quantity can reflect how the illness itself is progressing. Lastly, a trusted staff member may need to be called upon to communicate directly with the student on concerns surrounding problematic behaviors, along with suspected misunderstandings by the student of *other students'* behaviors and language. **Social Skills Groups** (as part of a speech and language program or counseling program) may also be warranted.

- Furnish Life-Skill Assistance

  The nature of the PANS illness can result in a profoundly *jagged* set of abilities that are needed to execute **activities of daily living**. (Such an evaluation may be obtained from an occupational therapist, among others.) If the student has regressed considerably from his peers, or if he suffers from lethargy or weakened fine motor or other abilities, he may need assistance and training in such areas as grooming, meal preparation, dressing, and transportation (including the use of public transportation), etc.) The goal is to furnish the student with skills that will help him *help himself* as much as possible, even during waxing periods of the illness.[3]

Organizational Supports

- Consider Preferential/Assigned Seating

  Such seating can lend itself to providing easier access to the instructor, specific materials, the exit door, or assistance when needed.
- Implement the Use of Assignment Notebook, Planner, Daily Assignment Sheets, Lists, and School Websites

  School or teacher websites can include present and future assignments, and in some cases, provide records of work that has already been completed and submitted. In addition, the use of a cell phone to record teacher dialogue and to take pictures of homework assignments listed on the overhead/ board should be considered.[4]
- Break Projects Down to Manageable Chunks

  Sometimes, students cannot see *"the forest through the trees."* At the same time, however, many of these students cannot see the *"trees for the forest"* either. For example, the student might glance at an assignment before her, and become immediately overwhelmed at what her gauge of the size of the work, or work product, will be. As a result, she may become frustrated and mentally 'give up' before she even gets started. In this case, the student may have difficulty *breaking down an assignment or project into workable chunks* that can be completed successfully, and in a timely manner. At worst, this inability can result in feelings of despair and frustration, even before an *otherwise capable student* begins her work.

  In these instances, pupils may need help with doing a **task analysis** of the work ahead. Projects and assignments can be segmented into smaller units, which can then be consecutively completed one at a time. Moreover, such a system will also offer positive reinforcement for work that they *have* accomplished. Binders with indexes that identify and break up sections can also be helpful. In instances where the student does not have the energy to do such a task analysis, the teacher or assistant may need to be proactive and do this for her.
- Prepare to Transition to The Next Class Earlier and/or Leave Specific Classes Earlier or Later

  Such modifications will allow the student more time to remember, organize, and collect materials and belongings for the next class, or when leaving for the day.
- ***Discreet*** Use of Cues/Prompts of What's Needed Next

  Whereas this line of questioning works well one-on-one, it is prudent *not to single out this one student* in a classroom for such questioning. If a teacher is going to do this, he or she should approach *a variety of students*. If the teacher remains concerned that the student is not following along, she might check with him after class as well (or touch base, of course, with the special education teacher, other related staff member, or parent).

- Implement a Home/School Communication System
  Communications via email[5] or notebook with parents can offer an additional layer of help regarding organization. Feedback can be exchanged regarding what is expected, received, or still needed. Moreover, many schools now offer the opportunity for parents to see current and future assignments 'on line,' along with what their student has turned in, or is still missing or incomplete.
- Provide Opportunities for SPED (Special Education) Check-In
  Periodic check-ins with the special education staff can provide additional help (for both the staff and student) regarding organizational strategies. For example, the special education teacher or assistant may assist the student in organizing his backpack and binders every Thursday etc. Moreover, the student may be able to keep organizational materials and relevant work, etc. in an area of the special education class, to be used later for other classes.
- Designate a Safe and Organized Place to Keep Belongings
  Sometimes, an assigned locker will not be practical for this student for a number of reasons. Sometimes it is too far away from classes, or it is located in an area where the student does not feel comfortable. At times, a locker may mean yet another layer of things that the student has to organize and remember. In any case, if another more convenient locker or storage place is available, the staff should consider that option. For many students, however, the special education classroom, counselor's office, or nurse's office will also serve as a safe place to leave a backpack, jacket, gym clothes, or other materials to be used during the day.
- Provide an Extra Set of School Books at Home; Color Code Books and Materials (that would assist in easy recognition of appropriate textbooks)
- Keep Extra Supplies on Hand (at home and school)
- Model Organizational Strategies, by Providing a Structured Classroom, and by Organizing *Distraction-Free* Study Areas at Home and at School such as the use of work carrels (TMI-*Not!)*
  "TMI" stands for *Too Much Information/Input.* We know that many of these students suffer from visual perception weaknesses. A visually 'cluttered' classroom or work area can be overwhelming, or at the very least, distractive to the student who is attempting to complete the tasks at hand.

Attentional Supports

- Implement *Organizational* Supports (as noted in previous section)
- Provide *Simple* Directions
  Obviously, it is easier to process one or two simple directions, than it is to follow multiple directions. Directions should be short, concise, and for some students, written down. Moreover, directions that are repeatedly used in a typical class can be written in a 'bullet' form on desks or on the blackboard. In instances where a student suffers from anxiety and has weak fine motor skills, for example, it may be of great source of comfort and support if he knows that *he can count on* seeing a daily work plan written on the board (and staying on the board) all day. In other instances, the student may not have the ability to *process* what is going on in the classroom, and *write down the daily plan* in a work book *at the same time*. As a result, 'note taking' is done *at the expense of his learning subject matter* or hearing important oral directions. A reliable written timetable that can be referred to at any time will reduce one of the many cognitive demands (and potential stressors) that this student will be faced with during his day.
- Consider Ear Phones to Block Out Distracting Stimuli
  Sometimes earphones may be helpful in blocking out distracting stimuli, especially when sound levels or sound types are perceived as disturbing. Alternatively, the task at hand (such as a listening activity,

or a recorded story) can involve the use of ear phones. In some instances, there will be students who will be able to complete a given activity more easily if they are listening to a preferred piece of music, set of sounds, or even '*white noise*.'[6]

- <u>Consider the Use of Study Carrels</u>
  As listed in the section above, these would serve to support attention by providing *physical boundaries* to the student's work area, thus blocking out unwanted distractions.
- <u>Provide Students with Flexibility and Choice in Selection of Work Stations</u>
  Whereas this can include priority seating in the class (next to a window, teacher, or in an area that is less loud or bright), it can also include the allowance for flexibility in body position, such as being able to stand to do work, or sit in a bean bag, or on the floor, etc.
- <u>Provide Positive Feedback For What They Are Doing *Right*</u>
  Like most of us, students do well when they receive positive feedback for what they're doing right. As these students descend into dysfunction, the more likely they will be to receive negative feedback, from peers, family members, and other teachers. They themselves may be very self-critical, as they begin to struggle in areas that were formerly non-problematic. *Honest feedback*- for what they are doing right- can be very validating and welcome amidst a sea of failed attempts and disappointment.

  At the same time, however, *too much* attention involving support/praise may be overwhelming for that student (especially if it is perceived as going above and beyond *what his peers are receiving*.) In this case, the instructor must be sensitive to a student's preference for not being *singled out* or "babied" amongst his peers.[7]
- <u>Allow for and *Encourage* Periodic Check-ins</u>
  Check-ins among the staff members, parents, and student, can help determine waxing/waning levels of attention as the illness progresses. In turn, this can allow for an adjustment of accommodations, instruction, and expectations, as needed.
- <u>Consider Levels of Stamina and Listening Skills</u>
  It is important to note that sometimes, poor attentional skills may be secondary to the sickness symptoms of the illness itself, to poor listening skills, or to other medical conditions (such as seasonal allergies, etc.).
- <u>Provide Opportunities for Breaks and Movement When Needed</u>
  Most human beings would undoubtedly think and feel better if they took a short break after forty five minutes of study, learning, reading, or writing. However, breaks become especially critical for students affected by PANS. Opportunities to move about, or even stand when needed, can help the student regain focus and attention. Sometimes the need to use the restroom or a request to take something to the school office can lend themselves to such opportunities. Moreover, an *Adapted PE* specialist can be called upon for ideas on quick exercises to use when the student feels that he is losing concentration.
- <u>Offer Opportunities for Students to Re-do tests, and to Demonstrate Knowledge of Subject Matter in Ways that may not be with Pencil and Paper</u>
  Can the test be given orally? Can the number of test items be reduced without jeopardizing an accurate gauge of his knowledge? Can he take half the test today and half tomorrow?

Behavioral Supports

<u>Part 1: General Considerations in Determining Types of Behavioral Supports</u>

- <u>Include *"Behavioral Supports"* as a Necessary Component of this Student's 504 or IEP.</u>

Provide clear **procedural safeguards** for teachers regarding the recognition, reporting, and management of unexpected or disruptive behaviors. The student study team (which should include input from the medical provider, parent, school nurse, and treating mental health provider) must work towards determining and clarifying the <u>*types, frequency, and severity*</u> of these behaviors, <u>as they relate to the student's illness and the ability to participate in the classroom</u>.[8]

At the same time, **it is of paramount importance to recognize that <u>*these behaviors are symptoms of a medical illness.*</u>**

As such, every effort *must be made* to accommodate for the student's disabling condition (PANS), by modifying the learning environment, and by adjusting the instruction, testing, and student participation, to whatever the student is capable of. When planning how to best adjust the environment to serve the student when problematic behaviors emerge, consider a wide range of interventions that can take place, both inside and outside of the classroom, and that are temporary, short term, or long term, depending on the student's needs. (Temporary interventions might include going home for the afternoon to rest, retreating to the library or to another place of refuge to study, or going to the 'computer corner' of the class to complete assignments on the computer.) Of course, a guiding principle is to strive for placements into *the least restrictive environment* that the student's disabling condition (PANS) will allow, (in this instance, as revealed by specific behaviors, *or even, lack thereof*).

When the behaviors become *chronically intense or disruptive enough* that they can no longer be accommodated for in the current learning setting, <u>***the team***</u> should consider another class placement that may be more appropriate (even for a limited period of time) until the behaviors wane. These may include provisions for home/ hospital instruction for all or part of the day, or a different classroom setting, or with a teacher who can offer more advantages for this student's needs, etc. In some instances, a more *"restrictive"* setting may be necessary, such as a resource class, a special day school, or a residential placement. (Also see the continuum of alternative placements in Section III).

- <u>Establish the Identity of a Trusted and Knowledgeable Liaison at School (a Counselor, Behavioral Health Provider, Nurse, or Guidance Services)</u>
  Such support systems within the school can be called upon to provide assistance, interventions, and strategies (including relaxation and specific therapeutic techniques) to be used at school and do at home.
- <u>Collaborate with Community Mental Health Providers as Needed</u>
  Similarly, a mental health care provider from the community may be called upon to participate as a valued student study team member, to offer guidance and input regarding the behavioral support of the student. Along with the student's medical providers, this 'outside' mental health provider is in an excellent position to elaborate on the etiology surrounding the student's behavior and learning ability. She is also in a position to validate efforts made by the student and family that have been attempted to address these concerns (whether or not they have been effective).
- <u>Consider that both the Therapeutic Treatment (and Efficacy of That Treatment) May Reflect a Paradigm Shift</u>
  PANS represents a distinct cluster of debilitating symptoms that include unexpected and inappropriate behaviors. Such symptoms directly result from the student's own bodily responses to infection or other triggers. Consistent with the waxing and waning nature of this illness, observed improvements (or regressions) in behaviors may sometimes be *mistakenly attributed to psychotherapeutic interventions*, when, in fact, improvements have been *due to changes brought on by the healing process of PANS itself*. Similarly, *treatments that have worked successfully with* other same-aged *peers with the same psychiatric diagnosis*, may *not always predict the same outcomes with* this *student,* especially if he is currently in a 'waxing' state of the illness.[9]

- Consider/Acknowledge/Document Waxing and Waning Nature of Behaviors
  To the extent possible, staff, along with the student, should become aware of how behaviors, alertness, and mood, wax and wane, often during the day, but especially over the weeks and months as the illness regresses and heals. In this way, modifications and supports can be increased or decreased as the needs change. (Also, in offering reflective feedback, the student takes *an active role* in his own healing and recovery.)
- Accommodate For Tic Symptoms as Needed
  When tic symptoms begin to interfere with full and active school participation, considerations must be made to provide refuges, breaks, and testing modifications. Self-help techniques, which may 'camouflage,' or lessen the severity of tics, etc. should also be considered. In collaboration with the parent, primary care provider, and treating therapist, the IHCP or Student Study Team can brainstorm both the triggers and management of tics. Sometimes tics that are viewed as socially inappropriate may result in the need to educate others regarding tics/PANS/Tourette Syndrome. In some instances, physical therapy may also be needed, in response to certain types of tic behaviors. For example, *repeated tics* can result in constant stress on certain muscle groups, and/or lessen activity levels.
- Accommodate for Mood Changes and Anxiety Symptoms as Needed
  As symptoms flare, a reduction of academic demands may be necessary. These can include a temporary reduction or elimination of homework, a *reduction* or *prioritization* of what needs to be completed on tests, and even a narrowed focus on what subjects are now seen as essential to maintain. These would likely include reading, writing, and arithmetic, and any topics that the student is still demonstrating success in. Consider *alternate* demonstrations of knowledge of subject matter from those that require pen and paper.
  Be cognizant that these students may be at higher risk for *not* attending school altogether *(school refusal)*, in that they may be experiencing feelings of failure, underachievement, and social isolation. It is true that these students may be especially sensitive to having attention drawn on them. However, to the extent possible and appropriate for their age group, show indications of kindness, care, concern, and support for their continued participation in the class, even if it is only for a few moments after instruction. Acknowledge *what they are still able to do*, even if it is only in their efforts to *still come to class*, despite their discomfort. Teachers should let these students know that they are available to talk, or to review class work as needed. Students should also know what other academic or counseling help is available in this regard. Other interventions that may be needed include a reduction of their sensory overload, the allowance for breaks and places of refuge, and relaxation and stretching exercises (that can also be facilitated by the teacher for the *whole class*). Lastly, it is very important that steady communication between the parent and teacher occur (if necessary, before, during, and after class) so that all can be kept abreast of the student's condition, and adapt and act accordingly. If the parent knows for example, that the student has had a difficult night with little sleep and worsening anxiety, she would do well to email, or otherwise contact the instructor or counselor, so that the latter can adapt instruction, or the student's work load, as needed.
- Accommodate for Obsessive Compulsive Symptoms, as Needed
  Assess the nature of the behavior (*what, when, where*), and brainstorm possible solutions. Allow for sufficient transition time between activities. For short periods of time as the student is healing, modifications regarding attendance may be needed to accommodate for morning grooming activities (such as tooth brushing or dressing) or other symptoms surrounding with 'nesting' behaviors, which may take longer than expected to complete. Such measures will allow for both psychotherapeutic, as well as medical treatments to take place that will eventually lessen the severity of such extensions.
- Prepare for Behavioral *Storms/Tsunamis, Meltdowns,* When Necessary

At their worst, PANS sufferers may become highly reactive, and possibly lash out. Of course, the best way to deal with such crises is to avoid them all together. An important way to reduce the number of these incidences is to recognize probable triggers that can result in high reactivity. In consultation with the student study team, including the school nurse and treating psychologist, arrangements can be made (beforehand) to address this type of eventuality. For example, the student might go to a designated place that is safe and calm, and where he can 'regroup,' if he or if one of the staff begins to suspect increasing overwhelm. (Perhaps there could also be a code word or phrase which can be exchanged among those necessary, so that this shift in activity will be as discrete as possible.) However, even when such triggers are identified, and contingencies like these are made, such behavioral *Storms* may not always be unavoidable. Meltdowns are often the strongest indicator that an individual is *feeling completely overwhelmed* by the surrounding circumstances or stimuli (whether *external* or *internal*), and is no longer able to self-regulate emotions and behaviors in response to such triggers. Whereas the likelihood is stronger that such meltdowns would occur at home rather than at school (or in public in general), the following considerations may nevertheless be useful if such events were to occur.

- Diffuse...Diffuse... Diffuse.

  If suspected sensory overwhelm may be a factor, aim to remove layers of sensory input (light, sound, movement, etc.) as much as possible and as discretely as possible. Sometimes, even direct eye contact can be too much for this student. Verbal communications should be brief, calm, and direct, and given from as few people as possible. Short directions (that access the logical part of the brain) are preferable to long commentaries and raised voices (especially regarding how he *should* be acting and what will be the negative consequences of his actions if he does not "shape up").

  Remember that when this student is in the middle of this neuro-behavioral *Tsunami*, he will be very much in the *immediate present*, in that ***he will be blind to the lessons of the past and any negative consequences that may await him in his future***. In such moments, he will likely be responding from the *fight/ flight* center of his brain, in which catastrophic self-narratives drive ensuing behaviors. Such behaviors are *purposely driven,* however, as the *brain is directing desperate attempts to self-protect.*[10] In such states, this student will have comparatively less access to the rational, prefrontal area of the brain (associated with critical analysis, etc.).

  With this in mind, as the student struggles to regain a sense of calm and self-control, those around him may be of greatest help to the student (and themselves), if they just remember to follow this one maxim:

The less this student has to cognitively process right now, the better.[11 12]

- *Develop an* ***Emergency Plan.***

  This should be part of an IEP, an IHCP, or any other educational plan, where anyone on the team feels that such behavioral storms may occur. Four important aspects of such a plan include the following:

1. *Consider The Probable Triggers Than May Set This Student Off, and Recognize Signs of Rising Overwhelm.*

Once a student is in the midst of such a *Storm*, he will have a reduced ability to fully articulate what is bothering him, or what has precipitated his reactivity. As a result, any explanation for why he is 'out of control' will likely not happen then, until he is 'back in control' (if even then).

2. *Designate a "**Captain**" for When a Storm Occurs.*
For those who are in the midst of this emergency, it will appear to be no less serious than a hostage situation, or a crisis on a submarine. As such, it will work best if there is only ONE person in charge. That person, and that person only, should be directing others (to leave with the other students, signal others to turn out lights, call for assistance, etc.).This *absolutely* is no time for those with differing views to negotiate what should be done.
As part of this protocol, the *Captain*, and/or assistants, should consider what *language,* or *phrases,* they will have at the ready, to explain- *briefly, succinctly, and directly-* to students, passers-by, and others, regarding what is happening, and what is being done to address the situation.[13]
Lastly, this 'Captain' may not necessarily be the lead teacher, but anyone who is in the *best* position to direct the situation, stay with the student, and facilitate what is necessary to bring him 'back to center.'

3. *Identify The **Connector,** or Entity, that Enables this Student Get Back to a 'Calm Place.'*
This may be the 'Captain,' but it also may be another trusted adult who is nearby. It may be someone who is available by phone who can facilitate the student's ability to calm down. Depending upon the student and the environment where the meltdown occurs, an animal, sibling, friend, therapist, relative, or even a distractive activity (such as **redirection** of activity or attention[14]) can facilitate a shift back to center. In some cases too, a policeman, an individual with medical training, or other 'authority' figure can help facilitate such a shift too. However, *diffusion* is still key.
When the child is ready and willing to do so,[15] he can then be asked very *simple and short* questions about his feelings and actions, which the listener might acknowledge by paraphrasing and repeating back for clarification. Similarly, verbally reflecting this student's feelings can also be soothing, ("So, when ________ happened, it was really frustrating for you. Would it help if next time, we______________?"). Most importantly, assure that the student is in an environment where he feels safe and supported, and where he can be given time and space to 'regroup.' Typically, the student will know when he is ready to re-engage.

4. *Find out, and put into place, related safeguards in accordance with medical, legislative, an organizational requirements.*
This is especially important in the possible event of physical aggression, or threat to bodily harm to self or others. Any selection of appropriate protection strategies and techniques must carefully balance clinical, safety, and security requirements.[16] [17]

Part 2: Special Considerations Regarding Behavioral Health Treatment

- Therapeutic Techniques
  A number of therapeutic techniques may be helpful as students grapple with the management of their illness. Some of the more commonly cited anachronisms related to specific treatments include **CBT:** *Cognitive Behavioral Therapy*, **ERP:** *Exposure and Response Prevention,* **ACT:** *Acceptance and Commitment Therapy*, and **DBT:** Dialectical Behavioral Therapy. Moreover, providers often work with individuals to learn skills in **relaxation**, **meditation**, and **Mindfulness**[18] techniques. ERP is often used as a standard treatment for Obsessive-Compulsive Disorder (**OCD**). ACT and DBT are also used as modalities in the treatment of anxiety, mood, and other disorders, and can be of use when one is suffering from chronic pain or discomfort.

Both ACT and DBT use components of 'Mindfulness,' which is a technique that focuses on the ***non-judgmental awareness*** of what is happening in the moment. It is the learned ability to become aware of one's discomfort, thoughts, mood, etc. in the moment, without the immediate attachment of meaning.[19] For example, in the case of a youth with PANS, this might be addressing a ruminating narrative of automatic disaster that is tied with specific triggers (like a drawer that is not closed in a certain way). In effect, the very exercise of Mindfulness can add a critical layer of cognitive support (coming from the rational part of the brain) that will, in turn, help this student navigate his actions when under stress. Instead of the "Ready, *Fire!*, Aim" mechanism of a behavioral Tsunami then, (where a child feels overwhelmed by his circumstances and immediately erupts), he can learn tools to access that logical, rational part of the brain (needed to observe, reflect, and articulate). Then, he can immediately access such tools *the moment he starts to sense discomfort.* With the help of a trained therapist, perhaps he can learn to practice this technique first by focusing on something that has not triggered upset. Through the use of such tools and others, he can learn over time to first consider the *"aim"* part of the "Ready, Aim, *Fire!*" process, and hopefully (with the intercession of his budding frontal lobe) avoid the *Fire!* part altogether.

- <u>Consider That Some OCD Behaviors Can Be Moving Targets</u>
  Some behaviors may wax or wane over time, along with the illness itself. In addition, often times behaviors may diminish, only to be replaced by new behaviors.
- <u>Acknowledge Logistical Concerns</u>
  As discussed in the first section that focuses on health supports, the act of traveling can at times be difficult, stressful, and even dangerous for students affected by PANS. In these situations, it would be helpful to consider a meeting place closer to the home, or where the student attends school. Alternatively, consider comforting entities that might accompany the student on the trip, such as a pet or a distracting hand-held game. Other alternatives surround the instruction of the parent and teaching staff in the use of appropriate therapeutic techniques and phrases *that they*, in turn, can help the student to use. At the very least, assure that preferential seating in the car is provided.
- <u>Note Differences in Medication Response from Non-PANS</u>
  As noted in the work of Dr. Tanya Murphy and her colleagues, youth with PANS tend to be far more sensitive to certain neuropsychiatric medications[20] than their same aged peers.[21] In this regard, providers, parents, and appropriate school personnel should discuss possible side-effects of prescribed medications, which may also include supplements. It's important to keep in mind that some care providers may not associate certain behaviors or conditions with being potential side-effects of medications, especially in medications for children.
- <u>R/O Post-Traumatic Stress Syndrome over Time</u>
  The intense nature of the PANS experience may also make those most closely involved with this student suffer symptoms consistent with PTSD. Even as the illness itself is in remission, consider that those with close ties to the student may still be sensitive to the same triggers that previously affected their student (and by extension) themselves so profoundly. At the same time, as healing progresses and symptoms diminish, caregivers should be provided support and opportunities to slowly disengage from heightened levels of focus towards this child.
- <u>Recognize Different Perspectives as Valid</u>
  Perspectives expressed will be heavily influenced by cultural, gender, socio-economic parameters, and developmental/maturational factors, as well as cognitive impairments brought on by the illness itself.
- <u>Consider HIPPA Protections and Limitations Regarding Access to Information (US)</u>[22]
  A clear concise understanding of what can, (and cannot) be conveyed to other family members and to the student is necessary to avoid breaches of trust. Moreover, family members must understand that in compliance with child protection laws, physical or other types of suspected abuse must be reported to authorities.
- <u>Consider 'Behavioral' Types of Therapies (as well as any prerequisite skills needed for their implementation)</u>
  According to Dr. John March, a leading psychologist in the use of Behavioral therapies, the application of **Cognitive Behavioral Therapy (CBT)** provides a number of advantages. He notes, for example, that

OCD is resistant to traditional insight-oriented psychotherapy, and the benefits of behavioral psychotherapy, such as in the use of ERP, are well established. Dr. March includes the following as key elements in the use of CBT for the treatment of OCD, for example:

- Keeping the focus on OCD as a neuro-behavioral disorder,
- Providing a graded **Exposure and Response Prevention (ERP)**, that is guided by the child's selection of targets,
- Implementing a "tool kit" for managing dysphoric affects and faulty thinking habits; and
- Providing psycho-education for family members and school personnel (as team allies).[23]

At the same time, Dr. March cites the following *factors that will determine the effectiveness of this type of therapy*. Predictors of success include the *presence of overt rituals*; the person's *desire to eliminate symptoms*, the person's *ability to monitor and report symptoms*, and the person's *willingness to cooperate* with treatment.[24]

In other words, for this treatment to work, the young person must have the developmental, cognitive, and emotional readiness to effectively participate in such therapy. In instances, therefore, where the youth *has* received such treatment, but has not yet demonstrated the hoped-for changes in his behavior, consider the possibility that the *waxing* nature of the illness has reduced his ability to observe process, reflect, evaluate, and remember certain events. Give therapy another attempt when symptoms start to wane, or consider scheduling sessions during times when he is typically more rested and calm. Especially, consider the age and the level of impact the illness is placing on the student before jumping into a specific therapy. In the onset of severe and debilitating PANS' symptoms, even older students may have difficulty engaging in various therapies. (At the same time, consider that even when students *lack the ability to demonstrate* self-calming and other techniques presented in therapy sessions, this does not necessarily mean that they have *not learned, stored, and remembered these techniques*. It may *only mean* that *other elements* are still barring them from implementing these techniques when needed.)[25]

As with any other person pursuing help through psychotherapeutic counseling, there is no one-size-fits-all protocol. Also consider other therapies and interventions designed to reduce stress level responses in general, such as exercise, yoga, and meditation.[26] Other treatments that involve forms of acupressure, such as **EFT**, have also been helpful in reducing a fear-heightened emotional response in individuals.[27]

Still another promising tool includes the practice of **Mindfulness meditation.**[28] [29] Psychiatrist Dan Siegel describes Mindfulness as an "integrated state of mental processing that involves a wide range of attentional, emotion regulating, conceptual and observational processes that are harnessed in a flexible and adaptive manner." [30] Of special significance to students with suffer from such limitations temporarily brought about by PANS, Mindfulness meditation, defined as 'being aware of one's sensory experience in the present moment,' has been shown to improve a number of processes that support physiological, mental, and interpersonal domains.[31] [32]

Additional Behavioral Health Considerations:

- Consider the Concept of Pain and Discomfort as Being *Real* for the PANS Sufferer

  It is important for caregivers to be aware that for many students who suffer from PANS symptoms, their pain and discomfort, especially in regards to sensory overload, *is very real to them,* and virtually indistinguishable from any other kind of physical or psychological pain. In these instances, validation and acceptance for how they are feeling may be the first step in enabling these youngsters to move forward toward acceptance and/or treatment.

- Grab Teachable Moments When Student Is Rested or Illness is Waning
  Perhaps the bulk of such therapeutic work could be scheduled during the times the illness is waning. Perhaps this student can attend therapy, but for shortened periods of time, on Skype, or at times of the day when he will be more alert and receptive.
- Explain the 'Brain Basics' of PANS to the Family and to the Student
  To the extent that it is appropriate and understandable for the listener, talk about the roles that the Limbic System, Prefrontal Lobe, Basal Ganglia, and Brainstem play in everyday life. Explain how PANS can challenge brain function associated with mood, attention, fine motor skills, etc. Include the ways in which brain function can be helped by appropriate treatment.
- Include the Family as Participants, and Include Parent Training
  In this way, perhaps the parent could introduce or reinforce relaxation techniques, Mindfulness, or other techniques, as instructed by the therapist.
- Encourage Writing Activities
  Research has acknowledged that the very act of writing about experiences, including unpleasant ones, can have a positive effect on the healing process. Gratitude journals and other types of writing activities can not only be therapeutic, but also foster better writing skills.
- Provide Opportunities For the Student to Have a Voice
  Once a student is jettisoned into the throes of PANS, he will likely have fewer opportunities that signal a sense of independence and control over his life. Often, the hours of his days are governed by the dictates of medical, educational, and other advisements and constraints. He may face constrictions on where he can go, activities he can do, and foods that he can eat. His day may be further punctuated by timetables dictating when medications must be administered, and when and how lab tests must be done. At the same time, he may see younger siblings and peers have expanding freedom and privileges to explore *their* environment, and expand their social community.
  In these instances, it may be helpful to determine those opportunities for control, that the student *can direct and determine*. These might include participation in a hobby, club (such as Boy Scouts) obtaining a pet, choice in a summer or school break activity (including staying at home), or having a say in simple decisions, such as giving him different food choices, or selecting different options, (including timetables) for the completion of an activity that is of low interest to him.
- Explore Web Resources For Cognitive Behavioral Therapy
  Whereas the gold standard for this type of treatment steers toward working face-to-face with a qualified therapist, there are also a number of web resources for CBT, relaxation techniques, and other therapies that can offer simple tools[33] to use, in conjunction with prescribed techniques, or in instances where in-office therapy is not possible.
- Consider Relaxation Techniques
  Such techniques can easily be brought in to general and special education classrooms *for the entire class* to use as a resource. Such activities can include deep breathing exercises, stretching, and other short activities that can facilitate relaxation responses for all students.
- Consider Home Visits
  Similarly, in instances where in-office therapy appointments are not feasible, home visits by a therapist can make treatment possible. Therapy appointments, especially arranged during times of transition (such as in the mornings and evenings) can actually provide instructive opportunities for the therapist *to see* the difficulties that the student is having first hand (i.e., slow grooming, eating, interference from siblings, transitioning to bed time, etc.). The therapist would then be in an excellent position to problem-solve and to formulate solutions that will work for that particular student (and in that particular home environment).

Moreover, in instances where the student and family are in a crisis situation, a home visit by the therapist can provide critically needed intervention, and in some cases, eliminate the need to call the police or fire department. In such instances where there is a bond of trust and respect that has already developed between the therapist and young person, the therapist may be in the best position to now facilitate self-calming techniques and tools taught in therapeutic sessions. (Such emergency intervention can also allow parents and other family members to have a much needed respite, even if it is short, in another room.)

- Promote Exercise!
  With diminished energy and stamina levels, participation in outdoor activities and group sports can lessen considerably among these students. Yet, the benefits of exercise on mental health, physical health (including the immune system), and cognition are well known. For example, we know that among other things, exercise helps to build up long-term memory, and also strengthen the hippocampus.[34] To the extent possible, the student, as well as the entire family, should exercise to maintain stamina and well-being.

Sensory Supports

- *Auditory* Overload or Distraction
  Consider the use of carpeting, lowered ceilings, tennis balls on chair legs, acoustical tiles that diffuse or absorb sound, P.A. systems muted or turned off, and headphones, ear plugs, or other protectors. Also rule out oversensitivity from positive (or negative) feedback that involves loud or repetitive speech, or other types of sounds. Care must be taken to both *solicit and allow the student to express his need for a quieter environment.* Therapeutic listening activities, such as the formal programs *Tomatis*, *Berard Auditory Integration Training (AIT),* and *SAMONAS,* have also been used to help individuals with auditory sensitivities.[35]
- *Visual* Overload or Distraction
  Consider the use of muted colors in working areas, and the use of blinds and curtains as needed. Consider the use of natural lighting when that amount is sufficient, and monitor the use and effects of florescent lighting, computer use, and other types of lighting on behavior and stamina. Reduce visual clutter in work areas and classrooms (as these students may have difficulty with selecting salient or relevant visual information out of a larger field of visual information). Certain 'Light therapies' and colored lenses have also been reported to help with both light sensitivity, and also types of cognitive dysfunction.[36] Lastly, strategically placed furniture can provide visual boundaries that will limit distraction and visual overload.
- Rule out Olfactory and Tactile Stressors
  It is important to consider that some of these students may also be affected by particular odors, chemicals, or fabrics. In these instances, identification and avoidance of such stressors can reduce overall levels of sensory overload.
- Consider the Use of Occupational Therapy Evaluations and Related Recommendations to Help with Sensory Overwhelm
  Sensory Integration theory originates from the work of Dr. Jean Ayres, who was an occupational therapist. Based on her experience and research with children, Dr. Ayres put forth the theory that sensory integration is the organization of all of the "sensations to move, learn, and behave in a productive manner".[37] Those OT's who have been trained in sensory integration **(SI)** can help identify and remediate areas of sensory integration dysfunction in affected individuals. SI also addresses difficulties with sensory overwhelm (to light, sound, movement, etc.).

Memory Supports and Executive Functioning Considerations

- Reduce Stress/Anxiety/Distractions as Much as Possible
  All of the above can thwart the ability to retrieve and relay information effectively.
- Reduce Cognitive Demands/Loads During Waxing Periods of Illness
  - Reduce or eliminate home work.
  - Allow time and personal space for this student to settle into the class, prepare his materials, and execute work.
  - ***Do not call on this student***, unless you *know* that he is attending to what is going on, and you feel confident that he knows the answer. (Questioning to determine if the student is *"really paying attention"* will be counterproductive for this student, and worse, will temporarily exacerbate his learning and memory difficulties further.) In instances where the student suddenly appears to be confused after being called upon, paraphrase the question, and give him a choice of several probable answers.
  - Focus on 'high stakes' classes and material, such as mathematics, reading, and writing skills. Other subjects may need to be of less focus now.
  - Provide structure, so that the student has one less cognitive demand that he must negotiate.
  - Give him notes or copies of the overhead material that is to be covered in class.
  - Give concrete and clear examples of what he is expected to know for the class and for the test. This can include highlighted material in text or notes.
- Teach Organizational Systems that Are Simple, and at His Developmental Level
- Provide Direct Instruction to Student in Memory Aids
  These can include *mnemonics,* such as PAR (Picture It, Associate It, Review It) or HOMES (around the Lakes of Huron, Ontario, Michigan, Erie, and Superior). Such strategies will help solidify and/or help in the recall of prior knowledge.
- Incorporate a Review and Repetition of Material into Instruction
  However, in instances where directions are going to be repeated back to the instructor, the teacher must be mindful to have *various* students repeat the directions back, instead of just focusing on this one student.
- Present Only as Much New Information as a Student Can Handle at One Time
  In this regard, look for visual cues that the student is at "saturation point" and/or overwhelmed. It might be time for a break or change of activity. Such changes in activity levels can include going from sitting to standing, or changing the type of learning activity to include moving or interacting with others.
- Provide New Information Within a Meaningful Context
  Associating tasks that are focused on areas of interest, or at least surrounding areas of accomplished competency, are to be encouraged, as they will better link new information with what the student already knows.
- Help Students Identify Their Areas of Strengths and Weaknesses
  Each student will have areas of strength that will prevail, regardless of where he is at in the disease process. Whereas many students with PANS may have visual processing skills and processing speed weaknesses, for example, they may have retained good auditory processing and verbal memory skills. As much as possible, the student himself should learn to become aware of these prevailing strengths, so that he can draw upon them when needed.
- Allow for the Use of Calculators, Math Facts Sheets, Digital Tape Recorder, Smart Pens, and Lists, etc.

The use of low and high-tech memory supports will be indispensable to assist students with short-term, long-term, and working memory difficulties.

Fine Motor Supports and Considerations

- Extend Time for all Tasks Involving Writing
  This would include handwriting, typing, the use of manipulatives, and all learning activities and projects that require eye-hand coordination.
- Provide for an **Assistive Technology** Workup/Assessment
  As part of an IEP, 504, or an IHCP, an assistive technology work up/evaluation would define the parameters of need, as well as determine appropriate technology, that would help accommodate for this student's needs.
- Allow for the Use of a Note Taker and Recording Equipment for Lectures
  These may also be needed for any other activities as well that require note taking and participation.
- Consider Shortening Long Assignments (such as every other item, prioritizing work, etc.)
- Consider the Use of Oral Responses, a Scribe, or Recorder for Test Responses, etc.
  Investigate the use of voice recognition software to provide speech-to-text capabilities.
- Provide Multisensory Support
  For students still developing their handwriting or cursive writing skills, extrasensory support involving tactile and visual cues will be helpful. Such support can include raised lined paper and ridged boundaries for handwriting, etc.[38]
- Consider Occupational Therapy
  An occupational therapist can provide appropriate evaluations and recommendations regarding fine motor difficulties, and related difficulties. They may also be able to rule out difficulties secondary to sensory integration problems, etc. An Assistive Technology specialist may also want to collaborate with the OT regarding appropriate recommendations for this student.
- Foster the Instruction and Play of Musical Instruments when Stamina Allows
  In addition to facilitating cognitive growth associated with the development of musical skills, the playing of musical instruments can support the development of manual dexterity. Depending upon the type of music and the student, the playing of music can also have a calming effect.

Gross Motor Supports and Considerations

- Provide Adapted PE/Physical Therapy, with an Emphasis on the Student Maintaining as Much Daily Movement as Stamina Will Allow
  Even in instances where the student may not be able to fully participate in daily PE classes, recommendations should be made by related staff to promote and facilitate as much movement and ease of gross motor ability as possible through sports and other exercises. Moreover, opportunities to exercise during the day may be needed to mitigate hyperactivity/agitation.
- Provide Assistance/Monitoring on Field Trips
  These students may need extra assistance in negotiating unfamiliar or unleveled types of terrain, and going for outings that involve long walks. Related considerations on field trips include the monitoring of stamina and hydration.
- Assure That There is Sufficient and *Proactive* Playground Supervision

Such supervision and interventions are necessary to promote fairness and access to physical activity and recreational sports. (This is in addition to assuring that all students are able to participate in recess activity without fear of being harassed or threatened.)

- Arrange for OT/PT and Adapted PE Recommendations Related to All of the Above
  To help in instances where students demonstrate difficulties with balance, coordination, and movement,[39] an OT, PT, and/or APE teacher could offer appropriate evaluations and interventions.

Speech and Language Supports and Considerations

- Rule out Hearing Loss or (Temporarily) Impaired Hearing (from ear blockages, etc.)
  These would include congestion from illnesses or allergies.
- Evaluate for the Need for Speech Therapy
  Such an evaluation would rule in (or out) the need for help in the areas of language *expression* (involving the articulation and intelligibility of words) and language *comprehension*, which includes the understanding of utterances, and that also include the processing of body language. Also consider and rule out the presence of sound sensitivities.[40]
- Provide for Listening Activities to Support the Development of Language [41]
- Consider Participation in Social Language Groups
  Such groups are facilitated by speech therapists and others to model and foster appropriate language skills in social groups and activities.
- Consider the Need for OT /or Speech Therapy
  Such therapy may be needed to improve (or manage) hypersalivation, dysfluency, and tic related utterances/movements, along with the management of sound sensitivities.
- Teach The Student Appropriate Phrases; Role Play
  This can be especially helpful to improve social language or to have language 'at the ready' if frustration, difficulties, or need for assistance surface.
- Consider Adapted Music Lessons and/or Music Therapy[42]

Visual Processing Supports and Considerations

- Consider an Auditory "Interpreter" For Movies, Videos, or any Learning Activity that Involves Sustained Attention and Visual Memory
  Just as individuals who are blind, or have low vision, may need someone to interpret movies and other images, those students who have weak visual processing speed may need someone to review visual information that is changing rapidly (like instructional videos, plays, news casts, etc.)
- Consider Maintaining a *Verbal Focus* on Instruction
  Sometimes, the presentation of visual information *along* with auditory information may slow down one's ability to process the instruction effectively. Be aware that the use of *multisensory* teaching techniques, in this case, may not always be the most effective. *(On the other hand, remember that not all students with PANS will have difficulties with Visual Processing).*
- Preview (with the student) Visual Material to Be Taught (Through Handouts, Discussion, Outlines, etc.)
- Differentiate the *Teaching* of *Learning Strategies and Cultural Practices* (including Social Language/Pragmatics) from How This Student *Actually Processes Information*
  Most students, especially at the primary grade levels, rely heavily on their *visual sense* to learn new information. This is reflected in the teaching of most pedagogy surrounding this age group, and is obvious to any visitor who glances upon the walls of most elementary grade classrooms. However,

the students affected by PANS may have needs that, once again, don't fit so neatly into the usual teaching methodology for his or her age group. These often problematic instructional strategies can include typical adaptations, such as those that emphasize visual processing, or multisensory strategies adapted to serve 'most' students (including those with dyslexia or other special needs).

Also, *look to the eyes*. Sometimes students may not be able to both LOOK at a speaker, process facial and body movements (including the meaning of those movements/gestures), AND process auditory information simultaneously. If she is looking out the window during instruction, for example, one must not automatically assume that she is "tuning out," "being disrespectful," or is otherwise disinterested. Keeping her eyes elsewhere may be *the only way* she can actually process what the instructor is saying. (Alternatively, it is also important to be aware that in some cultures, looking directly at an authority figure is deemed inappropriate.) In any case, if the student is constantly looking elsewhere during instruction or conversations, the provider or parent may want to address this with the student (in a way that is perceived as exploratory in nature.)[43] In some situations, the student (or parent) may need to take the proactive role in confirming with the speaker/instructor that he or she is listening, but does better using their auditory processing only.

- <u>Consider the Accommodation for More Time on Most Tests and Projects</u>.
- <u>Reduce Visual Clutter in the Classroom and Work Space.</u>
- <u>Consider the Use of Blinds, Curtains, Muted Colors, Natural or Full Spectrum Lighting, Clearly Defined Colored Boundaries, and Sunglasses When Needed.</u>
- <u>Rule out Visual Processing Sensitivities.</u>
- <u>Implement Recommendations as per OT/Developmental Optometrist.</u>

  These can include periodic eye exercises and the use of eyeglasses. If the student is not wearing his prescribed glasses on a regular basis, attempt to determine why, in order to problem solve solutions.[44]

Part 2: Supports Related to Academics: Math, Reading, and Writing Skills

Considerations Specific to Math

Math Supports I

- Share Data Validating *Extra Time f*or Tests (Requiring Memory, Fluency, Fine Motor, Attention)
  Math instructors, like any other instructors, need to acknowledge that extensions on test times and other accommodations are *based on verified data,* that *has determined a clear need* for such measures. Therefore, *it is not* under that teacher's discretion to decide if, when, or where to provide such accommodations. In some situations, with the consent of the student and/or guardian, the principal, psychologist, or special education teacher may want to explain *why* there is the need for accommodations (such as the student having weak fine motor skills, etc.). This can be especially helpful in instances where the math teacher has not attended the Student Study Team meeting. However, *it is not required* for modifications and accommodations to be implemented.
- Provide Explicit Training in the Use of Assistive and Organizational Devices
  These can include the use of graph paper, weighted pencils, and computer programs, and the use of such technology as *Bookshare* (that will download textbooks) and *Livescribe Echo Smart pen*, etc. that will record aspects of presentations, etc.
- Include Computer Software in Regular Education and Special Education Classrooms that Provide Supplementary Instruction and/or Practice in Math Concepts
  Of course, this must be used with prompting, supervision, and instruction from a *qualified teacher*. Such programs can accommodate for memory, organizational difficulties, and the need for extra time to consider responses, etc.
- Shorten Assignments
  Again, the focus should be on obtaining competence in subject matter and demonstrating sufficient knowledge to reflect this competence. In this regard, one must be clear about what exactly would suffice *to demonstrate competence* for the student. For example, does the student actually need to do twenty-five problems to demonstrate competence in his ability to subtract single digit numbers? Would seven items suffice? Shorten assignments (and tests) where multiple items are evaluating the same skill. Remember, the longer the math assignment or test is, the greater demand there will be for *sustained attention, working memory, and short-term memory*. Therefore, the greater risk there will be for burn-out and decreased productivity over time.
- *Prioritize* Assignments on Homework/Test Items
  Similar to that discussed above, in collaboration with the teacher, parent, student, and special ed. staff, decisions can be made to confirm the Top Ten or Top X number of items that need to be done to show mastery of subject matter. On some nights, the student may have limited ability to complete all of his work. What are the *most important items* (and *number* of items) that the teacher feels are needed to show participation, learning, and mastery?
- Provide Breaks
  Secondary to the above, breaks, at least every hour for ten or fifteen minutes, will allow students to disengage or regain energy before going forward. Moreover, work completed in segments will also allow opportunities for mental and/or physical breaks. Perhaps even more importantly, though, they will allow for a sense of completion and achievement for the student, as they now complete workable chunks of tasks. For example, an agreement can be made for the student to just do the first four items, take a break, and then complete another four items, etc.

- Allow for Dictated Responses
  Poor fine motor skills can pose obstacles in the student's ability to write equations and graphs, and to solve subtraction and multiplication problems, etc. Can the instructor confirm mastery of subject matter if she or an assistant *verbally queries* the student on how to solve a given math problem? On math tests, can the use of computer programs that use multiple choice formats, calculators, and speech-to-text be used? Could the student, for example, select the correct formula to use when solving a statistical or algebraic problem, out of a field of five different formulas, etc.?
- Encourage the Use of Mnemonics
  (GEMDAS) Order of Operations (**G**rouping, **Ex**^{2}, **M** (×), **D** (÷), **A**dd, **S**ub) is an example of a mnemonic that serves as guidelines and reminders to students in a particular subject matter, such as math. Mnemonics can be devised by the teacher or created by the students themselves. (The goofier and/or 'racier' the mnemonic, the more likely it will be remembered.)
- Track Math Scores as Much as Possible
  For many of these students, math scores may wax and wane along with other symptoms of their condition. In addition to considering fluctuations reflected on chapter tests and report cards, *standardized measures* of math abilities (completed in earlier school years) can usually be obtained through the School Districts.
- Allow for The Use of Math Facts, Formula Sheets, and Calculators (Including 'Talking' Calculators)
  The use of such low-tech and higher-tech items can be helpful and appropriate when this knowledge is not the primary purpose of the test.
- Consider Dictation and/or Scribe
  In instances where fine motor skills have substantially reduced the ability to write numbers, formulas, and equation, etc., the instructor/ team should consider options whereby the student can verbally explaining the solution, with another writing the numbers down.

Math Supports II (Instructional and Placement Considerations)

- Consider Activities that are *Teacher-Directed*
  In a teacher-directed style of instruction, the teacher models the mathematical procedure to be used, and then checks for understanding before moving on. In this way, the teacher is assured that she is *only adding on one new element* to what the student already knows. As much of math instruction and learning is scaffolded around prior knowledge, it is important to confirm that the student has already mastered any prerequisite skills, before moving on to new concepts. In addition, a review of the steps may be periodically needed.
- Facilitate Self Questioning and Self-Monitoring Strategies
  One example includes the use of check lists, whereby the student can check off items as they are completed before proceeding in his work. This can also provide a sense of mastery and self-control, which in turn, supports self-esteem as well.
- Provide One-on-One Tutoring as Needed
  This may be necessary to supplement instruction at school, or it may be provided through home/hospital instructional programs. One-on-one tutoring is often the best way to accommodate for significant memory and attentional weaknesses. In this situation, the tutor or instructor is in an excellent position to get immediate feedback as to whether or not the student is staying alert and comprehending concepts, through their body language, verbal responses, and other behaviors. As such, she can then immediately adapt or accommodate her instruction or the activity, as needed.

- (Re)Consider the Use of Manipulatives
  Manipulatives are tangible items that, in this case, are used to represent mathematical concepts. An example of a manipulative is a ***Cuisenaire* rod**, where one block represents a ten-digit value, another a hundred-digit value, etc. The use of such items can be helpful, but they need to be used with caution. This is because any impairment in eye-hand coordination, memory, and attentional skills can thwart the ability to manage these items effectively, thus rendering them of questionable value as learning tools.
- ***NEVER Decide On Advancement/Retention of Math Level Based on One or Two Data Points***
  PANS symptomatology will likely affect test results and homework quality throughout the duration of the illness. Advancement or retention of a math level should be based on a *variety of measures* over time, and not just one or two tests at the end of the term or year. If there is *any question* as to the student's competence, a math specialist from the school district, or someone from outside of the school (who is impartial to any outcome) should work with the student to determine current math skills and readiness levels.[45]
- Provide Routine Clarification with Staff Regarding Modifications and Accommodations.
  Is the math teacher clear on what the modifications or accommodations are for this student? Does the student and/or special education liaison signal that these are implemented on a consistent basis? If so, *how* are they being implemented? (In another room? Over the course of several classes? On a computer? Dictated to the student on a blackboard or overhead?) Moreover, is the teacher or other staff sensitive to how, when, and where the accommodations or modifications are implemented? If the student is given extra time on the test as an accommodation, for example, how does the staff assure that this overtime won't run into his recess time (that he also needs to refresh, regroup, and/or to get to another class)?
- Carefully Consider any Implementation of On-Line Math Work or Courses
  Such work can be a great asset, in instances where fine motor, memory, and organizational skills are affected. Computer work completed in the classroom can also offer students options for staying in a *least restrictive environment,* while keeping up with math lessons (at a pace that works for them, and where they can get immediate (and *discreet*) feedback if the response is, or is not, right). That said, caution is in order when considering the implementation of on-line math *courses* (especially) at *higher levels of math*, such as Algebra and Geometry. Very generally speaking, unless the student is truly passionate, competent, and diligent about doing math work, he or she will need someone *physically* there to model procedures, check for understanding, and monitor progress on a consistent basis.

Considerations Specific to Reading and Writing Skills

- Consider the Use of Assistive Technology
  Assistive technology will aid in the processing, use, and demonstration of literacy skills. When the processing of text is slowed by weakened visual perception, consider such text-to-speech technology as *Kurzweil*, *Bookshare*[46] and other programs, that have the capacity to 'read' textbooks and other printed material (and that are free to all US students who qualify). Consider the use of speech-to-text programs that will enable students to dictate writing assignments and test responses. Consider also the use of recording devices such as *Live Scribe Smart* pens that will record presentations, etc.
- Provide Extra Time to Process Texts, Tests, Homework Projects, etc.
  Just as extra time in mathematics should be a major consideration when processing speed is compromised, so it should be for the completion of reading and writing assignments. At the same time, it is also important to acknowledge that for many students, *such extensions may accumulate*

work for the student as time goes by. Especially for those students who struggle in these areas, the accumulation of unfinished work may result in high stress levels for all concerned, particularly as the end of the semester or term approaches. Here, the student may begin to associate schoolwork with failure, frustration, and hopelessness, as he learns that despite his best efforts, he will only become progressively more behind as the term goes by and peers move further ahead. Similarly, attention must be given to how a possible lag in the submission and completion of such course work will bear on his grasp of subject matter; that is usually needed as a base for the understanding of future lectures.

- Include an Accommodation To Write *Directly* on the Test Protocol
  This accommodation is helpful in instances where memory, attentional, fine motor and/or organizational skills can thwart the ability to go from test protocol to answer sheet. As one processes material from one sheet and then formulates the answer to its test questions, sometimes it can be difficult to transfer and place the correct response on the appropriate place on a second answer sheet. In these instances, it may be easier for the student to just circle the correct response on the (original) test protocol.
- Consider Shortening or Modifying Assignments
  Again, without compromising the actual skill, standard, or level of competence to be mastered, instructors should carefully consider what parameters need to be met to indicate mastery. As described in the math section earlier, can the student write fewer examples of a particular standard or skill to demonstrate mastery? Or, can this knowledge be demonstrated in portfolio collections of work, where this knowledge is demonstrated in a variety of submitted work? Could the student do *every other* homework item, or can the work be prioritized, with the top ten items needing to be done first, and with other items done if the student has sufficient energy?
- Consider the Use of Dictated Responses on Tests or Other Activities
- Eliminate Crosswords, *Hangman,* or Other "Fun" Puzzle Type of Assignments
  The majority of such "fun" assignments puts incredible demands on sustained attention, fine motor skills, visual processing, and memory, with the resulting product yielding little 'payoff' for such exacting efforts and time. Unless expressly requested by the student, avoid these types of exercises and test items. Design and connect written class work, homework, and test questions to explicit content, skills, or tasks that need to be mastered instead.
- Introduce Mnemonics
  SQ3R (Survey, Question, Read, Recite, Review) and *HOW* (Heading, Organization, Writing) are examples of mnemonics that can serve as guidelines and reminders to students in their Study skills and writing and reading assignments. Again, such mnemonics can be devised by the teacher or created by the students themselves.
- Incorporate Mental and Physical Health Activities
  As these students regain their health, the inclusion of literacy activities that will also support physical and mental wellness can be very beneficial. Such activities can be especially helpful in circumstances where periods of alertness and ability are limited during the day (and at *certain* times of the day). Such activities may include **journal writing** as they progress from illness to wellness. Other activities may include **gratitude journals** and **charting of behaviors**. Still other writing assignments (perhaps surrounding particular aspects of PANS) can be used to develop skills of critical analysis and perspective. Last, but not least, consider books of interest (either read or listened to) where students can see themselves in the struggling hero who prevails over former difficulties.[47]

Universal Design for Learning and the PANS-Affected Student

Universal Design for Learning (UDL) is a concept that serves as a guidepost to address the unique learning needs of all students. Specifically, UDL endorses the following provisions that work to ensure that every student, regardless of level of ability or disability, is afforded a fair and appropriate education:

- **The Offering of Equal opportunities** to learn.
- **The Implementation of Flexible approaches** to instruction (and demonstration of mastery of skills) that can be customized and adjusted for individual needs.
- **The Provision for Multiple means of Engagement.** This surrounds the "Why" of learning, and surrounds aspects of recruiting interest, sustaining effort and persistence, and student self-regulation.
- **The Provision for Multiple Means of Representation** This entails the "What" of learning, and would surround the aspects of perception, language, expressions, and symbols and comprehension.
- **The Provision for Multiple Means of Action and Expression.** This addresses the "How" of learning, and entails such aspects as physical action, expression, communication, and executive function.[48]

Inherent in its design, and of special relevance to students with PANS, UDL works to ensure that a number of important educational considerations are taken into account. First, its design addresses the often regressive, halting, and jagged nature of cognitive development and achievement in affected children. Next, it acknowledges that there are, in fact, *multiple continuums* of service and need (as opposed to a *'one size fits all'* service model for all students with special learning needs). Moreover, UDL promotes the notion that 'Special Education' is not 'a place,' and that assistance should occur in the most appropriate and least restrictive environment. Last, but not least, UDL acknowledges the many ways that mastery of academic standards can be demonstrated.[49] For example, in some instances, criteria to meet standards in *multiple subject matters* can be met in the submission of *one project*, where all such competencies are addressed.

What might this look like in practice? The following is an example of how, in collaboration with the teacher, parent, and perhaps the student's therapist, a seventh grade student could work towards the mastery of a number of skills in one such project (as reflected in the standards below).

Reading and Writing Standards for Literacy in Science/ Technical Subjects- 6-8th Grades

- Reading Standards: Obtain key ideas and details from text, and integration of knowledge and facts.
- Writing Standards: Involve informative exploratory texts, short research projects to answer a question (including a self-generated question), drawing evidence from informational texts to support analysis, reflection, and research.
  (California Department of Education-Curriculum Framework and Instructional Resources Division, 2011)

A Sleep Study by Dolores Frazier 11/5/2015 - 11/19/15

- Date: Sun. 11/5/15 Wake time: 8 am
- Number of minutes of exercise I completed today: 0
- Activities during the hours before bedtime? Played Little Mermaid videogame.
- Bedtime: 9 pm

- Date: Mon. 11/6/15
- Wake Time: 7am
- Duration of sleep last night (From bed time to wake time:) 10 Hours = 600 minutes
- Number of times awakened at night: 4
- Number of min. awake after going to bed: 80 Subtracted from total? 520
- **Total minutes** in bed **asleep** (estimated): 520 Percentage of Total? 520/600 = 86%
- Quality of Sleep I had last night from 1-10 (with 10 feeling fully refreshed): 5
- Possible factors in changes of sleep quality last night?: *(Levels of light and noise, pets, exercise, worries, bedtime routines, discomfort, relaxation techniques/ other therapies, new medications/ supplements, bed or blanket issues, foods, temp., etc.)*

  Bedtime routines (teeth brushing), worries, noise in other room

  ____

- What will I do tomorrow (or next week, etc.) to make (or keep) improvement? (e.g.) I will stop playing video games within 2 hours of going to bed./ *(or)* I will start getting ready to bed at eight./ *(or)* I'll try the relaxation technique that my counselor told me about (etc...)

  (Abbreviated Charts designed with symbols indicated AM/ PM, etc. can be marked off or circled easily. Graphs can show daily/weekly results and findings.

The types of questions in the chart above can be used as a springboard to develop and demonstrate competencies across the curriculum. Moreover, such projects can also encourage analysis, reflection, and self-help skills regarding the student's healing process. In conjunction with a fill-in type of chart like this, a student could develop a simple 'Monday through Friday' chart that could also be ticked off quickly in the morning or evening. In accordance with the reading and writing standards listed above, the student could easily incorporate her research of facts and figures into a design of a chart and a "Write-Up" (or "Results") section. Information investigated could include the effects of sleep on health, and the effects of specific factors on the ability to maintain sleep, (such as lighting, diet, lack of exercise, noise, worries, etc.). Notice also how math skills may be easily incorporated into an assignment like this. In this case, percentages are focused on. However, depending upon the skill level, addition, subtraction, Algebra, or statistical computations may be implemented. In addition, a 'Mood checklist' could utilize words, faces, or write-ins to describe how the student felt on a certain day or how he felt about himself on a certain day.

Part 3: The Important Role of Assistive Technology

Undoubtedly, for most people, the use of technological aids (such as computers and cell phones) has made life much easier and more efficient. However, for most students with disabilities, and especially for students with the debilitating symptoms of PANS, the use of technology can make the difference between getting through school, *or not.*

Assistive Technology (**AT**) can play a significant role in assuring that all students have fair and full access to as many aspects of their education as possible. Some of the more common applications of assistive technology serve to facilitate the following:

Instruction

Whereas 'in-person' teacher to student instruction is still considered to be 'the gold standard' for imparting new information, there is a surge in the use of technology designed to make instruction accessible to learners who may have difficulties with comprehension, memory, fine motor, attentional, or visual or auditory limitations. Recording devices, such as *'smart pens'* allow for the audio recording of lectures that can later be repeatedly listen to as needed. Even today's cell phones have the capacity to record visual and auditory information from the class, as well as capture notes from overheads and blackboards.

Student learning that is gleaned through reading and writing activities can be facilitated by a variety of assistive technology devices. Programs such as *Bookshare* (offered free to US students) and other programs such as *Kurzweil* \ *Victor reader*\and *DAISY* [50] offer the opportunity for text and other books to be highlighted in the text, and "read" to the student (text-to-voice technology).

Of special importance to one's ability to remember and synthesize what has been read, this 'reading' is at an *understandable speech rate*, (in contrast to the often slowed reading rate that results from weak processing speed). This is important, because, as the slower reading becomes, the more that student will have to rely on his short-term memory and attentional skills to recall and synthesize the passage. *'Reading Pens,'* too, can scan text, which is then downloaded and then 'read' through the computer's text-to-voice program.

Still other computer instructional programs can facilitate and support learning by identifying skills already mastered, by providing feedback to students on their work (in a safe non-public way), and by reinforcing self-regulation regarding work that is completed and unfinished. Last but not least, the use of assistive technology accommodates the learner in terms of the learning environment he needs to be in (such as at home or in the hospital) through the use of *Mobile Tablets* and *e Readers*. Moreover, technology that can be used anywhere, such as *laptops, iphones, or ipads* can also provide Interactive type of systems, such as email, texts, *'YouTube'* related downloads, etc.

The Measurement of Student Competence

It is important to separate *the measurement of* a student's knowledge of subject matter from her *ability to demonstrate that knowledge.* For example, the student may know the material, but if she needs twice the time as others to finish the test due to the constraints of her disability, her scores will not reflect her true competency, unless she is provided extra time. Today's technology can make a huge difference to level the playing field in this regard. Speech-to-text programs such as *Dragon Dictate* and others can efficiently put spoken words into print that will be readable to others. With the manual entry of a few letters of a word, *'Word Prediction'* programs, such as those offered by *Kurzweil* and *iOS,* can cut down writing time by automatically filling in the rest of the word's letters. When demonstration of knowledge of subject matter is impaired by difficulties with spelling and grammar,[51] programs through *Kurzweil and Ginger*, etc. can make appropriate suggestions for corrections. Other programs allow for test responses to be manually entered or spoken directly into a computer. Similarly, when writing activities are impaired by organizational difficulties, programs such as *Inspiration Software* and others can help with the organization and execution of written work.

Obtaining Appropriate Technology

As the use of assistive technology will play a critical role in this young person's educational survival, it may be helpful to consider the following:

- Consider having an AT assessment for the student, provided by someone knowledgeable about such technology. Each student has unique needs, and different abilities and level of interest, that will affect how they learn and use such technology.
- Remember that rights to AT (and training programs to access this technology) are safeguarded under federal law.[52]
- Keep in mind that there are a number of free or low cost webinars on AT, where one can also learn more about the latest technology that's available.[53]
- Information is available regarding what programs are accessible in the local area and state wide.[54]
- It is recommended that products are tried before being purchased. Many of the more expensive programs (like Kurzweil, etc.) allow for a trial use. Some can also be borrowed or accessed from school districts, libraries, or other agencies.
- If students need assistive technology in the classroom, there is a high probability that they will also need this technology for such 'high stakes' tests (such as the **SAT**'s, or other measures that will determine class, college, or other placements). In this regard, make sure that both the need AND the use of specific accommodations have been documented, as these will be needed to obtain accommodations from testing agencies.

Part 4: PANS and Postsecondary Education

A New Set of Assumptions and Expectations

In the experience of many families, especially in the United States, the notion of *what is considered requisite* to initiate services and support for students appears to change the moment their student steps into a postsecondary school setting. In common practice, the most glaring difference between the two systems of education is that at the postsecondary level, the student *does not need to be failing* to receive help. Whereas under both 504 and IDEA legislation (at K-12 levels), students *do not need to be failing to receive accommodations* or services, the experience of many parents at this younger grade level is that they are often told that support is not necessary, *"because their child is keeping up,"* or is not at risk of failing his or her grade level. Of course, the parent or teacher may be quite aware that the student is only *"keeping up,"* because she spends three times the amount of time her peers do when completing the same work, and because the family is spending money on outside tutoring and other supports to facilitate such efforts.

At the college level, postsecondary institutions adhere to guidelines set forth by state and federal legislation, such as Section 504. Under these parameters, a student *can* and does receive services and accommodations if she has a documented learning disability, a medical condition, or a psychological condition that warrants accommodations or modifications. Again, this is true- regardless of *whatever* the student's grade point average has been, or her ability to "keep up" with other students.

Transition Planning in the *Pre-* Postsecondary School Years

If the student has struggled with PANS symptoms while still in high school, that secondary school can play a pivotal role in facilitating a smooth transition to the postsecondary level. Specifically, the counselor and the special education department should assure that as much as possible, the student has the necessary information and documentation that will allow him to have continued access to services and accommodations. Indeed, if the student has an Individualized Educational Plan (IEP), transition counseling is an integral part of the IEP planning. This includes surveying possible postsecondary school placements (possibly followed up by family visits to the hoped-for schools), as well as other postsecondary options that may not be academic. It could also include such things as learning to navigate bus lines, and to engage in other services that would afford the student greater independence, mobility, and access to the community.

Obtaining Services and Help at Postsecondary Level

In the case of a college student, the student himself, and hopefully his parent or advocate, would arrange to meet with the **DSPS** counselor (or equivalent) at that school. DSPS stands for **Disabled Students Programs and Services**. Every postsecondary institution that receives federal funding, and most private institutions, has some equivalence to this type of office. A learning specialist at the school may be called upon to help design an educational plan too. The plan would be based upon documented symptoms and need, and result in accommodations and/or modifications that could be implemented in the classrooms or other educational settings.

To obtain accommodations or modifications under 504, most colleges require documentation from the treating medical provider, psychiatrist, or other examiner who provides the diagnosis, along with an explanation of its educational ramifications for the student.

Documenting a Disability as the Result of a Medical or Psychological Condition (vs. a Specific Learning Disability)

At the college level, the process of obtaining accommodations and modifications for someone with a medical condition (such as PANS), compared with someone who may have a *'Specific Learning Disability,'* can be very different. For some, it can sometimes be perceived as less cumbersome.

Similar to what one would expect to happen at younger grades and age levels, if an individual is requesting accommodations for help based on having a learning disability or intellectual disabilities, the family or school is expected to provide findings of a comprehensive diagnostic evaluation. This includes, at a minimum, test results of cognitive/ processing functioning and 'achievement.' (The former includes such measurements pertaining to fluid reasoning, visual-spatial processing, short term memory processing, etc. Test results of 'achievement' would include such areas as math, writing, reading ability and comprehension, oral language skills, etc.) The student's fine motor skills, gross motor, and social skills are typically reviewed as well. The evaluation report must also include background information (including a medical and educational history), and a 'summary' section. Most critically though, the examiner must carefully *tie back* the test results with any proposed accommodations, in order to justify their use. For example, a basis, or **rationale,** for providing extended time, may be associated with the student demonstrating *slow processing speed* or *slow fluency* on tasks completed during the evaluation. Postsecondary schools, like other educational institutions, also require that the evaluation is conducted by someone trained and certificated in this area, such as a Learning Disabilities specialist, neuropsychologist, school psychologist, educational psychologist, or other expert.

Sometimes, students with PANS do bring documentation of psycho-educational assessments that confirm a **DSM**[55] or other prior diagnosis indicating a specific learning disability, or of some other condition, along with its ramifications on learning and participation in the educational environment. Such evaluation reports can be very helpful, especially if they demonstrate that the student has already shown evidence of both *need and use* of accommodations at earlier levels of their education. If students have such documentation that was completed in high school, for example, it is often sufficient *"to get the ball rolling"* towards obtaining services in college, (or in requesting accommodations for College Placement Exams, such as the *SAT*). (One caveat to this is to assure that the testing used was standardized, or normed, on adults, and/or was deemed appropriate to be used on that age group as well.)

However, even in cases where the student *has not had* psychoeducational testing, it is not impossible to receive help or accommodations for his or her disability. It is possible to obtain assistance, based on the affecting medical or psychological condition alone. Each postsecondary institution has forms, usually obtainable on their web sites, which can be filled out by the treating psychologist or medical provider. Such forms serve to document the medical and/or psychological condition, and detail how its symptomatology can affect and limit the student's functioning. Again, it goes back to tying the *evidence of the disabling* condition with the *need for* whatever *accommodations* that are being requested. For most students with PANS, the student would look to the medical provider, for example, who would indicate specific aspects of illness that would create barriers for her to be tested fairly in a typical testing environment (under normal timing constraints, etc.)

These application forms are usually about three to four pages long. Along with statements by medical providers or treating psychiatrists/ psychologists, it is also helpful to provide other supporting documentation too, such as that provided by treating occupational therapists, educational therapists, and binocular vision specialists, etc. For example, the occupational therapist may show the results of standardized measures of handwriting ability, where writing ability is impaired to the point that it is necessary for the student to have either a scribe for the writing for tests, or voice-to-text technology. Another type of testing that can be helpful in this regard is called the **ImPACT Serial Testing.**[56] (Whereas this last test is typically used to determine any cognitive changes (such as slower reaction time) in those who have suffered a concussion, it has also been normed on a group of patients suffering from a type of encephalitis, for example, too.)

In summary, the process for obtaining services and accommodations at the postsecondary level would generally be as follows:

- Review DSPS policies beforehand (usually available on the school's website).
- If applicable, review these protocols with the counselor at the student's high school (preferably in the spring of Senior year) to assure that all paperwork pertaining to accommodations and services are in place.
- Meet with the college DSPS counselor (preferably in the spring or summer prior to enrollment) to confirm and discuss accommodations and services. (If DSPS requires updated testing, they will

usually implement accommodations taken from K-12 documentation until updated reports are received.)

- Check in with the DSPS counselor (or college learning specialist if applicable) periodically to review status and effectiveness of accommodations and services, etc.

PANS and College Entrance Examinations

For students who are still in high school who are applying for accommodations on such College Entrance examinations, such as the **SAT**, etc., all of the types of documentation listed above are typically requested by their prospective agencies too (such as the *College Board,* etc.). On these types of tests, the most common accommodations and modifications include such things as having extra time on tests, a screen reader or a human reader, a scribe or keyboard entry aid, a separate testing room, a calculator or/and extra breaks.

Before asking a physician or other provider to fill out these forms that document a medical disability, (including forms for the *College Board* or *Educational Testing Service*, etc.), it can be very helpful to obtain the advice from counselors (either from the student's high school, from the local school district, or from the prospective college) to help navigate this process. (In the US, another valuable resource for adults with suspected or identified disabilities (in general), is the Department of Vocational Rehabilitation, a governmental agency that offers support to those with disabilities, in efforts to secure employment or training towards employment.)

To Test or Not to Test?

In some colleges, especially Community Colleges, testing is sometimes offered by Disabled Students Programs and Services, (or their equivalent) to determine whether a student meets the criteria for having a Specific Learning Disability (SLD). However, unless the student has an SLD, testing may not be necessary, or even useful. Interestingly, for many of these students in terms of test scores only, it is very likely that results of most standardized psycho-educational assessments would yield a substantial discrepancy between high verbal ability and/or high reasoning skills- and their (most likely) weak processing speed and slow academic fluency. This could then (on paper, anyway) possibly translate into students requiring accommodations, for more time to complete work, etc.

However, in this case, the disability is secondary to a *medical condition*, rather than to a 'specific learning disability' per se. In addition, as with younger students who are affected by PANS, considerations must be made regarding the youth's levels of attention and energy, which may affect the outcome of testing. Moreover, as with the testing of a younger student with PANS, there has to be general acknowledgement that the student's present levels of performance are only a current "snapshot" of ability. Certainly, however, the college learning specialist might still be a valued resource in suggesting various college services that might be appropriate for that student.

Common Accommodations and Support Offered at the College Level

As one of the top accommodations offered to this student, **priority registration** offers the opportunity for the student, LD specialist and/or the DSPS counselor, to consider classes (and in effect, instructors) that would present a "best fit" for the student's needs, and then to enroll him in those classes before the general student body has access to such courses. Other common college accommodations that should be considered for this student include: **extra time on tests** (usually time and a half, but sometimes also double time), **voice-to-text** and **text-to-voice technology**, **access to assistive technology (and related instruction)**, such as in the use of *Kurzweil*), **course substitutions** (in cases where that knowledge is not essential to the student's major), the **use of a note taker, tutoring services, counseling services, testing in a distraction-free room, and mobility and seating considerations**.

The Notion of Full-Time Status If the symptoms of PANS are affecting the rate in which students can complete classes in a timely manner; this should be documented as well. If the college student is receiving a scholarship or other funding based on full-time enrollment, investigate whether a modification can be considered (on the basis that the medical condition requires the student to take fewer classes or units per semester). If no modifications can be given, encourage the student to include classes that don't require as much studying and effort, especially during the first semester. Also, be sure to include physical education classes such as yoga, dance, swimming, etc. in the course load.

The Parental Role and the PANS-Stricken College Student: (Yet another New Set of Assumptions and Expectations)

The role of the parents, in navigating and assuring the implementation of educational programs on their child's behalf, changes dramatically once the child is in postsecondary school. Actually, this can happen even earlier if the child turns 18 before graduating from high school.

Of course, with such a disabling condition as PANS, it is not uncommon for most students and parents to have spent months, and sometimes years, being "joined together at the hip" to assure for the most optimal academic outcomes. Therefore, it can be a rude awakening for parents to discover that they now need to be "invited" by their "adult" child to participate in any meetings or conversations regarding his educational fate. Yet in the US, from the age of 18 (at the latest, depending upon which state the student resides in), at least two sets of legislation come into effect, that bar any access or exchange of information regarding the student without the student's written consent. **HIPAA**, which stands for the ***Health Insurance Portability and Accountability Act***, basically outlines rules of confidentiality and privacy regarding medical, psychological, and other information. Most people are familiar with HIPAA guidelines through forms they have signed at their doctor's offices. Similar to HIPAA guidelines, **FERPA** stands for **Family Educational Rights and Privacy Act,**[57] and pertains to privacy laws of students in publicly funded post-secondary institutions. In their adherence to FERPA laws, secondary institutions have strict mandates surrounding the exchange of medical, educational, financial, housing, and other information concerning the student. These institutions will have various types of consent forms, however, to release such student information (i.e., **Consent to Release Information Form**). As students, families, and schools are now obliged to adhere to the mandates of such legislation, it is important that students understand and allow for such releases, *before* it becomes necessary.[58]

Students Now Assume the Mantle of Their Own Educational Fate

It is not uncommon that if a student has a disability as severe as PANS, a parent will either call, or come in to speak with someone at DSPS to elaborate on their child's medical status, educational history, and perceived needs. At the same time, families need to know that *in the classroom*, however, the student will usually be expected to be *his own* educational advocate.

Moreover, there will not even be any communication between the staff at the school's Disability Services center and the student's teachers, unless the student himself initiates it. The student must now *self-advocate.* He must let teachers know of any accommodations that he is entitled to, and provide the teachers with any documentation from the DSPS office, if necessary. If the student has received similar services sometime during his K-12 experience, the idea of broaching the topic of his educational needs with instructors may not be so intimidating. If self-advocating is new to this student, however, the DSPS counselor or LD specialist at the college should definitely review and rehearse *specific language/phrases* to use with teachers and others, for this student to have 'at the ready.'

Privacy Considerations

Students should also be made aware that teachers or professors do not need to know *anything* about their medical condition, or even what *aspects* of their cognitive function or processing abilities are affected. They *only* need to know that the student has a **verified disability** that allows the individual to have specific accommodations, etc.

Moreover, the student should also be made aware of the fact that, although he is afforded certain accommodations and modifications, that this does not mean he needs to use them for each and every class. He can use them solely when he thinks that they are needed.

Lastly, at the college level, as with any other level of education, students should be assured that there are instructors who will generally be understanding and helpful- if they know that accommodations will help their students demonstrate their true knowledge of the subject matter. (*This is where having a good and knowledgeable college counselor comes in*- one who knows *which staff members* will be best at implementing accommodations in respectful and effective ways.) Ultimately, however, it will be up to the students themselves, to decide how, or what, they want to disclose to staff and others about their condition, and how much they want to use the accommodations, etc.

PANS and Graduate School

As noted in their stories, many students with PANS have, at their core, some of the 'brightest minds of the bunch.'[59] As they heal and begin to reverse the regression caused by this illness, innumerable opportunities begin to open up, becoming real options once more. One of these is Graduate School.

For those students with waning PANS symptoms who are now reaching the level of graduate school, they should be encouraged to work with DSPS staff regarding accommodations for the **Graduate Record Exam,** and for other exams for entry into graduate level programs. If the student does not have a history of being served in the educational setting with documented accommodations, etc., already in place, he will have to provide medical documentation and other information (that was cited earlier for obtaining such accommodations).

And While We're Still on the Subject- **Additional Considerations Regarding The Postsecondary Level Experience: A Breath of Fresh Air for Many of Our Students**

For most students, there are increased intellectual, academic, organizational, and attentional demands that greet them when they step foot onto the grounds of postsecondary institutions. However, such institutions can also provide a breath of fresh air, and a new beginning for many of our students too.

As one proceeds further along on the academic escalator, the less one generally needs to do well in a *variety of subjects*, and the more one can zero in on areas that *one is strong in*, and are of true interest. Moreover, especially if one is afforded *Priority Registration*, one can begin their classes at times that best suit his or her own internal clock and health needs (as opposed to, for example, 8 am every day). There are also opportunities for taking longer breaks *between* classes at the postsecondary setting. Also, students are often allowed the option of taking classes at night, on one day a week, during the summer, or even 'on line,' etc.

Last, but not least, if the postsecondary school is larger than the high school the student has just left, (or if it is in a different area from her home town) this student may discover a new group of friends, and a new social network and community over time. Her fellow students will embrace her and accept her for who she is *right now*, and will be benignly indifferent to whatever 'baggage' or history, she has now (mercifully) left behind.

Closing Thoughts Regarding Accommodations, Modifications and Services

- Remember that these students can display *a JAGGED* presentation of abilities and achievement, both *over time*, and *within the same subject matter*.
- Remember that with appropriate treatment and effective academic support in place (including in *Advanced Placement Classes,* and *Classes for the Gifted and Talented)*, the trajectory and academic prognosis for this student is exceedingly positive.
- Acknowledge the need for an IHCP, a 504 and Special Education when called for, as well as tutoring, *Bridge* programs for Social Skills Development, OT, PT, speech and language, modified day, assistive technology, behavioral health, outside resources, home/hospital study, etc.

- Continue with periodic assessments, collaboration, and monitoring of ongoing services (such as OT and Speech and Language). Also, continue to monitor and clarify the *appropriate use* of accommodations and modifications with staff members as needed. Reevaluate the need for modifications and accommodations as symptoms wax and wane.
- Remember the legal and ethical mandates surrounding intolerance for bullying and harassment. Document and address such incidents as they occur. Discern a "safe" place, and a trusted, available staff member for the student to go to, should incidences occur.
- *"Teachers need to understand that they need more time to complete work and to 'get' new information."*[60]
- That said, *like anyone else,* these students too, must (eventually) take on the role of *primary agent* (and ultimate *owner*) of their own academic work and fate. Towards this end, providers, educators, and family members should consider ways in which they can help facilitate this ownership, by *'passing on the torch'* of responsibilities[61] to these students, whenever possible.
- Continue to recognize the *Authentic Person* within.

Notes

---

[1] *Outside agencies* generally refer to those service providers who are not part of the school district.

[2] As reported by providers and parents, sometimes changes in behavior as the result of food intake, can be difficult to connect, if children are reacting from food ingested earlier in the day and outside of the home. (Candelaria Greene, JF (2015) Unpublished survey of family members, providers, and survivors of PANS regarding PANS and Education (2013-2015), collected as UC Berkeley Visiting Researcher Scholar, Berkeley, California.)

[3] Some of the above support ideas taken from *Davis Unified School District, Farmington, Utah (from 504/IDEA comparisons)*.

[4] For many students, the use of such technology (as opposed to the use of a human note-taker) is preferable, as it is seen as being more *similar to what their peers would do*.

[5] Regarding email exchanges, as in voice mail exchanges, one must not assume that such exchanges will remain confidential. When in doubt, it is always prudent to be aware of all parties who have access to such communications (including anyone who might be walking behind the instructor's computer while she is reading the communiqué).

[6] *'White noise'* is a steady, unvarying sound, such as the sound of static on a radio or a television station with no signal. It is sometimes used to drown out other more bothersome sounds (like conversations going on in the next room while one is trying to sleep).

[7] A common theme noted by PANS survivors (Candelaria Greene, 2015).

[8] Sometimes, new and disruptive behaviors can be associated with unintended side effects of prescribed medications, which providers and parents especially need to be aware of.

[9] As noted by respondents (Candelaria Greene, 2015).

[10] Many thanks to Dr. Mary F. Candelaria, PsyD, Clinical Psychologist, Bellevue, W.A., for her insight and collaboration on the section surrounding mental health concerns.

[11] As psychologist Dr. Linda C. Avery astutely observes, during these times especially, students will "depend on the calming directive frontal lobes of others, until the *tsunami* passes, and they can regain the use of their own." (11/01/15).

[12] As Dr. Avery also points out, as this unfolding neuro-behavioral *tsunami* unfolds, it may be not unlike caring for an individual who is experiencing an epileptic seizure. The priority is *safety and support* within a *calm, trustful environment*.

[13] Such language might be something as brief as, *"We just need some space- We'll be out in a minute."*

[14] *Redirection* (of activity or attention) has been reported to be effective for some students with PANS (Candelaria Greene, 2015).

[15] Again, depending on the student, even the following line of questioning might be too much. Moreover, in consultation with the student's psychologist or treating provider, implementations of other procedures, or self-calming strategies (such as the use of *Mindfulness* tools) might also be considered.

[16] (The latter) advisement from *Caring for a person who is Aggressive or violent* from: Queensland Mind https://www.health.qld.gov.au/mentalhealth/docs/aggressive.pdf

[17] *Additional Thoughts Regarding Behavioral Storms/Tsunamis, Meltdowns:* Remember, once such a crisis begins to unfold, the lesson is no longer about '*Algebra*' or '*Dangling Participles.*' To be sure, these are (just) a few things that *every student who is witnessing this event* is now learning*:*

- Does The Person In Authority Act *Decisively, Calmly, and Confidently*, to secure the *safety of the student and others* in the class?
- *How Does (the) One in Authority **Treat*** an Individual who is not Behaving in Appropriate and Expected Ways? (Would onlookers want to be treated this way if they were in similar need? Is this occurrence being treated as other medical emergencies would be treated?)
- What is the *Effectiveness of the Behaviors* of the One in Authority on the Student in Question? Is the student able to calm down? Is he able to assimilate back into the class later on? Does the student become *more* reactive or despondent? *Does he not return to school-* perhaps out of fear or humiliation over this event? Does the one in authority show indications of braveness, kindness, and traits of effective leadership, etc? Do her or his actions result in the other students feeling secure, confident, and supported? Or, conversely, does the interaction leave the witnesses feeling upset, fearful, and/or sad for the student in question? (Has the student been yelled at, isolated, pushed, shamed, or threatened?)

[18] For excellent descriptions on Mindfulness and its applications, kindly see the following works: Daniel J. Siegel (2007) The Mindful Brain: Reflection and Attunement in the Cultivation of Well-Being, New York: W. W. Norton, and Jon Kabat-Zinn's (1996) Full Catastrophe Living (Revised Edition): Using the Wisdom of Your Body and Mind to Face Stress, Pain, and Illness. London: Piatkus. (Regarding the role of child development in discipline, also see Daniel J. Siegel and Tina Payne Bryson's (2014): No Drama Discipline: The Whole-Brain Way to Calm the Chaos and Nurture Your Child's Developing Mind. New York: Bantam.

[19] Thanks to Dr. Mary F. Candelaria (Interview June, 2015).

[20] Murphy, T. K., Storch, E. A., & Strawser, M. S. Selective Serotonin Reuptake Inhibitor-Induced Behavioral Activation in the PANDAS Subtype. Primary Psychiatry. 2006; 13(8):87-89.

[21] Peers who may suffer from the same psychiatric diagnoses (i.e. OCD) but who do not have PANS.

[22] Dr. Mary F. Candelaria, PsyD.

[23] From John March MD, MPH Program in Child and Adolescent Anxiety Disorders http://www2.mc.duke.edu/pcaad/abstracts/Integrated%20Treatment%20of%20Pediatric%20OCD.pdf (retrieved June, 2015)

---

[24] ibid.

[25] As reported by several PANS survivors, initial attempts at therapy to reduce stress levels and OCD symptoms did not seem to help; however, as they began to heal from the condition, and grow older, they noted that *they did remember* some of these techniques that had been taught to them earlier, and would often implement them- either on their own, or with the help of a therapist. (Candelaria Greene, 2015)

[26] For example, see a discussion of Daniela Kaufer's work in this regard, in Lehrman, S. (2008) *Nurture into Nature*: Meet Your New Brain. Cal Alumni Magazine Volume 119(2) March/April.

[27] For a better description of EFT (Emotional Freedom Techn que), please see Craig, G. (2011). The EFT Manual. Energy Psychology Press, Santa Rosa, CA.

[28] Such as that taught through the Mindfulness-Based Stress Reduction approach (Kabat-Zinn, J. (1990). Full Catastrophe Living: Using the Wisdom of your Body and Mind to Face Stress, Pain, and Illness. New York: Dell.)

[29] Siegel, D. G. Mindfulness training and neural integration: differentiation of distinct streams of awareness and the cultivation of well-being Soc Cogn Affect Neurosci 2007 2: 259-263.

[30] Ibid. p 261.

[31] ibid.

[32] Currently, there are grants and programs that evaluate the use of taking meditation and *Mindfulness* breaks in the classroom. In these instances, teachers or others take ten or fifteen minutes out of the day to practice these skills with students.

[33] Often, these can be available for free, as well.

[34] For a good review on this, see: Saadati, H., Babri, S., Ahmadiasl, N., Mashhadi, M.. Effects of Exercise on Memory Consolidation and Retrieval of Passive Avoidance Learning in Young Male Rats. Asian J Sports Med. 2010 Sep; 1(3):137-42.

[35] From Heller, H. (2002) Too Loud, Too Bright, Two Fast, Two Tight (2002) Harper, New York pp 201-206

[36] Ibid. pp. 207-219.

[37] Ayres, A. J. (2005). Sensory integration and the child: understanding hidden sensory challenges. P 5 (25th anniversary ed., rev. and updated / by Pediatric Therapy Network Los Angeles, CA: WPS.

[38] '*Handwriting without Tears*' is one popular handwriting program that incorporates multisensory strategies.

[39] Likely secondary to propioceptive and vestibular challenges (hypo/hyper).

[40] If in doubt, ask about this to the parent, student, and/or teacher.

[41] Listening activities are also available to support Sensory Integration as well.

[42] *Music therapy* is provided by a trained and certified music therapist to address *non-musical goal areas*, including speech, communication, social skills, motor planning, ills, etc. *Adapted* music lessons pertain to a modified approach of teaching music (such as signing, reading music theory, etc.). Such adaptations can include the use of visual aids or modified tuning, etc.

[43] In other words, in a non-judgmental way that assumes that the student is doing her best to participate in the activity or exchange, while providing important feedback to her on what is seen as appropriate or expected in most conversations.

[44] Consider the possibility, too, that the student feels uncomfortable wearing glasses around his peers. In this case, can contact lenses be obtained? Nevertheless, if neither the wearing of glasses *or* contacts is feasible for the student, offer the opportunity to sit in an area of the class that will offer better visual access, especially when if it is known that the diopter and/or astigmatism levels are high.

[45] This could be a math specialist from the school district or in a private practice in the community. It could also be a college student who tutors local students. The goal would be to just confirm current math levels.

[46] *Bookshare* is free under a federal grant that allows all qualified students to participate.

[47] Such as Michael Phelps with swimming and his early struggles with ADHD.

[48] CAST 2014. Used with Permission.

[49] Such as the *Common Core* State Standards in the US.

[50] Many of these programs offer free trials.

[51] (And when that knowledge (of grammar and or spelling) is not itself being measured.)

[52] These include such legislation as - Public Law 105-394 [29 USC 2201] of the Assistive Technology Act.

[53] Assistive Technology AMAC www. gatfl.org (Atlanta, Georgia) offers webinars on assistive Technology

[54] The Resna Catalyst Project (offers information regarding state programs.

[55] DSM stands for *Diagnostic Statistical Manual*, which serves as the handbook for the American Psychological Association. Identifiers for diagnoses and their associated Numerical Codes can be found in this manual.

[56] For more information, see www.impacttest.com

[57] 20 U.S.C. § 1232g; 34 CFR Part 99.

[58] FERPA has noted exemptions for the release of student information to parents. These include provisions for health and safety emergencies, if the student qualifies as a dependent (as defined by the IRS), and in cases where a student under 21 has violated any law or policy concerning the use of possession of alcohol or a controlled substance. For more information on FERPA see FERPA General Guidance for Parents (http://www2.ed.gov/policy/gen/guid/fpco/ferpa/parents.html)

[59] For example, histories of PANS' survivors include accounts of high academic success at the K-12 level, as well as at the college level. Moreover, despite the challenges posed by PANS earlier on in their education, some have gone on to attend such prestigious institutions as Columbia University and the University of Southern California. (Candelaria Greene, JF (2015).

[60] BG (PANS survivor; interview April, 2014).

[61] (However small the responsibility might actually be-)

Section VII

CLOSING COMMENTS

Signposts of Hope in the School Community

It is not to be overstated, how, with improved awareness of PANS,[1] most of the meetings, interventions, and strategies, etc. that have been presented in this book, *will simply not be necessary.*

With prompt and early treatment, any fluctuations of PANS-associated dysfunction will merely represent a possible 'footnote' on a student's educational history. **It is only when PANS remains unchecked,** due to a lack of diagnosis, *misdiagnosis,* or tragically, *no access to effective treatment,* that it will continue to wreak havoc through those precious developmental years. In these lamentable instances, PANS will indeed threaten to become a 'chapter' or 'major theme' in the young person's academic career.[2]

Like their non-affected peers, students with PANS look to their families and schools to help them navigate through their academic journey. Of course, such guidance and intervention becomes especially critical when regression, dysfunction, and other learning needs begin to emerge. In order to address the needs of students with such diverse and debilitating needs as PANS, then, where can schools and the governmental agencies that support them begin?

Practically speaking, there is only one way to serve students who manifest characteristics of such a paradigm-changing illness as PANS, where symptoms emerge, but follow their own timeline of regression and dysfunction. It is to have *good and effective* educational and special educational systems at the ready to address whatever the implications of the illness may be. In this way, it is fair to say that the degree to which a school responds to a PANS-*affected student,* can be viewed as the truest litmus test, for how that same school, or school system, would respond to *any student* who developed educational difficulties.

What then, may be considered positive indicators that the school *is* fostering and safeguarding the type of educational experience that will be *most appropriate* and *least restrictive* for this unique learner? The following questions and comments will help gauge the extent to which the needs of all students, particularly those with PANS, are being addressed and met.[3]

At the School Site Level:

a. How receptive is the school in their dealings with the family to ensure good and positive collaboration on behalf of the child? How is this receptivity demonstrated? How easy is it to exchange ideas with school staff, and to obtain information and needed services? How friendly is the 'front staff' (such as those in reception)?
b. Are staff members approachable and *accessible*? Can the family engage with school staff on a daily basis as needed? How quickly do they return phone calls? Can one come in personally and speak to the administration, counselor, teacher, special education teacher, or other staff member, after school, before school, etc.? In particular, what is the availability of the special education staff? Do they maintain consistent office hours? Are staff mindful and respectful surrounding issues of confidentiality? (For example, are they discrete and selective in their use of emails or other communications that may compromise privacy?)
c. Are staff members *proactive* in addressing the student's needs? (Do they notice symptoms at school and contact the home, or do they wait until they hear from the parent before they take action? Do staff members try to accommodate and adapt to students' needs *as they come up*, or do any interventions wait until they are *formalized* through meetings, etc?)

The School Administration:

a. How proactive and supportive are the administrators regarding the inclusion of students with special needs in their school, as well as the inclusion of *each* and *every* learner in their school community?
b. Do they communicate a collective and collaborative spirit when it comes to helping *all* staff members, and towards being a community of educators, support staff,[4] parents, and students?
c. Do they provide effective oversight of their facility and staff?
d. Regarding special education, accommodations, and modifications, etc., do they espouse, foster, and follow a set of guiding principles to ensure common direction among the staff?
e. Specifically, what do the administrators do to create an educational community that knows how to take steps to support students affected by PANS and their families? (Do they have staff meetings to develop an awareness of PANS and its education implications? Are teachers supported through funding to attend workshops on PANS? *Do they, the administrators,* take steps to inform *themselves* about PANS, or do they wrest this responsibility solely on the special education staff, or others?)
f. Do administrators (through grants or other monies) seek out and provide technology and related training, along with materials, equipment, and assistance from paraprofessionals, to correctly and efficiently implement services and accommodations?
g. Are administrators proactive in their stance against bullying and harassment, especially towards students with special needs? How is this stance demonstrated in their oversight and actions? (Do they provide workshops for teachers, staff meetings, disciplinary actions, student peer training, assemblies, etc.? Do they acknowledge and address taunting or bullying comments made by staff members?)
h. How creative are they in their ability to 'think outside of the box' in order to obtain additional services and support for students with special needs?
i. Do they acknowledge and account for the views of parents, teachers, the student, and other team members in decision-making? If so, how is this acknowledgment illustrated by their actions (at 504 meetings, IEP meetings, calls or 'check-ins' with parents, and informal modifications when needed, etc.)?
j. Do they take responsibility *for their role* in ensuring the delivery of a good educational plan in a *least restrictive environment*, as well as in the implementation of modifications and accommodations?
k. Are they respected among their peers and the staff they supervise?
l. Do they demonstrate knowledge and applications of education and special education law pertaining to their jurisdiction?
m. Do they encourage the collection of data and reporting that will allow for sound decision-making in educational planning and implementation?
n. Do they seek outside support and guidance when needed?
o. Do they acknowledge a lack of awareness in particular areas of expertise? When more information is needed, do they assume responsibility for finding out such information?

Educational and Planning Meetings:

a. Does the school consult with a registered school nurse for advice on educational plans that involve a medical condition (and where it is known that the medical condition can affect the student's education)? Do staff members understand that a School Nursing Plan is designed to ensure that the student's *health needs are supported* (so that he can participate in the learning environment as much as possible)?

b. Does the school staff demonstrate compliance with all applicable governmental [5] and other procedural safeguards having to do with timelines, etc.? (Do they meet or precede these timelines?)
c. Based on the guidance and parameters mentioned above, (as well as what is recognized as good and effective educational pedagogy), are policies and procedures provided at these meetings that will set the direction, clarify intent,[6] and guide coordinated work?
d. Are meetings held at a time that is feasible for both parents and other important parties to attend? Are out-of-district providers and others who are significant to the student's welfare, *welcomed and acknowledged* at these meetings? (Or, on the contrary, is there a feeling of secrecy and exclusion regarding who can participate at these meetings?)
e. Does the 'real' decision-making regarding interventions, modifications, and accommodations happen *at the meeting* and in response to the input of all parties, or in *advance of the meeting*?
f. Are participants introduced, and their roles at the meeting and in the planning process clarified?
g. Is the educational planning process itself clarified? Especially to new comers to special education, 504's, etc., are parents (and the student to the extent appropriate) given an explanation of what happens at these meetings? Are they provided with information about procedural safeguards and mediation, due process, and other avenues to pursue, if they do not agree with the services the school proposes?
h. Are resources available at meetings regarding PANS, and of its educational implications?
i. Are provisions in place to inform absent staff members about the proceedings of the meetings?

Testing and Assessments to determine the Need for Educational Services:

a. Does the school address ALL areas of need and suspected weakness?
b. Do they provide an assessment process appropriate to what the latest research indicates about PANS-related symptoms?
c. Do they consider fatigue and periods of waxing and waning that may affect testing results?
d. Do they suggest, provide, and pay for outside testing, when appropriate?
e. Are assigned evaluators qualified to assess areas of weakness (such as difficulties in visual perception, skills of daily living, and fine motor ability, etc.)?
f. Are testing norms based on what would be expected for peers (in the same grade, age, social, or cultural identity, etc.)?
g. Are changes or regression in 'higher risk' areas associated with PANS ruled out? These can include changes in fine motor and gross motor skills, behavior, level and types of movement, attentional levels, weight loss, eating habits, skills of daily living (such as grooming, bathing, etc.), mood, levels of fearfulness or anxiety, language, visual perception, energy, social activity levels, executive function, academic skills, and sensory response to light, sound, etc.)

Services and Related Interventions:

a. Has a school nursing plan been offered? If so, what kinds of interventions are indicated (based on her assessment of nursing needs and information gleaned through her interviews with medical professionals, family members, the student, and others)?
b. Is special education offered when needed, even if the student is maintaining good or excellent grades?
c. Are logistics taken into account when considering any 'outside' referrals for therapy, clinics, or other interventions?

d. When needed, does the team acknowledge and endorse the use of occupational therapy, physical therapy, speech and language, social skills interventions, counseling, adapted physical education, transportation, peer-support programs, etc? What provisions does the school have to obtain such services for the student when no in-house staff is available?
e. Are the parents aware that they can approve of the services and accommodation, etc. that are advised by the school, but decline the *placement* of where the services would take place? (In other words, sometimes, when parents visit the proposed classroom, they find that it would not be a good "fit" for their child, perhaps because of the needs of the other students in the class, structural barriers, or other factors. In this case, they may approve of the services, but not approve of the class placement.)
f. Are the *parents* provided with those services or supports necessary to assist their child in securing their educational plan? (For example, do *they* need counseling or training to help their child access technology, or behavioral supports, such as self-calming techniques, etc., in order to then support their child?)
g. If applicable, how does the educational plan address needs related to skills of daily living (such as grooming and eating) and any difficulties with executive functioning?
h. If present, does the plan include measures to address relief from sensory overwhelm (such as modifications in the classroom) and/or other types of overwhelm (such as providing refuges, etc.) that could interfere with the student's participation in school?
i. Are breaks, including breaks to go to the bathroom, arranged in such a way as to not draw undue attention on this student?
j. Are safety needs of students, teachers, and staff given *the top priority*? (Are emergency plans considered when needed?)
k. Are transition plans in place to guide the student in goal setting, and planning for the future?
l. In what ways does the team support the student in having as much *agency* as possible in her own education and welfare? (How does the team recognize and encourage, through their behaviors, language, and educational plan, the fostering of student empowerment, responsibility, decision-making, and control in that student's own educational journey?)

Modifications, Accommodations, and Special Educational Considerations:

a. Is the focus on this unique student, or is the educational plan based on a 'boiler plate' of 'typical' accommodations that are in place for 'most students with special learning needs?'
b. Are the accommodations and services directly tied to assessment results[7] (including those from the school nursing plan)?
c. What efforts are made to keep the student in a least restrictive environment? (For example, with support or modifications in the regular education class, instead of in a resource class or a self-contained special education class?)
d. What efforts are made to keep the student in 'Honors' classes, 'Gifted and Talented' programs, and 'Advanced Placement' classes? (Do team members understand that accommodations and modifications can be appropriate in these classes too?)
e. Has it been clarified to the staff members involved that any interventions are based on a verified disabling condition?
f. Do staff members acknowledge that the implementation of accommodations, modifications, etc. are *required*[8] and not just *suggested*? If so, how has this been communicated by the administration?

g. How does the educational plan acknowledge and address the student's need for *social* participation in the school environment? Do they acknowledge social development and participation as an integral piece of the student's education, that is to be fostered and safeguarded? How are needs related to participation at recess, lunch, and other activities *outside of the classroom* going to be met? (These can include field trips, dances, and participation at other school functions.)
h. Similarly, how does the educational plan foster and safeguard athletic activity and participation in group sports and teams, to the extent appropriate?
i. What indications are there that the staff implements interventions in *respectful, face-saving* ways to students? If tones, language, and behavior associated with the delivery of interventions or instruction are perceived as offensive, humiliating, condescending, negative, or non-constructive, what avenues are in place to address this?)
j. What kind of monitoring is available to determine effectiveness of interventions and strategies over time? (Who does this, how is this evaluated, and what is involved?)
k. Is **qualitative** feedback from parents, teachers, and students included in the reviews of program effectiveness? (In other words, in addition to quantitative measures that measure knowledge of math and reading with *test scores*, for example, are *qualitative* measures, that include subjective feedback from participants, included as well?)
l. If the educational team decides to assign a special education placement to a *Resource* room, (based on findings that the student is having difficulties with math, for example,[9]) is it clarified how *this* placement will address his needs *specific* to that subject?
m. Similarly, at the high school level, if the academic area of need is in math, and the team is suggesting a resource or special education class placement, does the special education teacher in question have expertise in teaching math at this level (algebra, geometry, etc.)?
n. How are testing accommodations (such as extra time on tests) supported in a way that the student does not miss out on instructional, recess, or lunch time?

The 'Regular Education' Classroom and Teacher:

a. Does the regular education teacher demonstrate an understanding of what the education plan is, and how it needs to be implemented?
b. Is the teacher supported in her work with students with special learning needs? For example, does she have adequate assistance, technology, etc?
c. Are *all of the* students in the class able to receive adequate attention and instruction?
d. Are interventions and accommodations provided in a natural 'non-spotlighted way' whenever possible? Are accommodations (such as extra time on tests) offered to anyone who needs extra time on work?
e. Is the teacher able to manage class members in the classroom and on the school grounds who may taunt this student because of PANS-related symptoms? If difficulties arise in this area, what is the school and educational team plan of action? Is this reflected in the educational plan when needed?
f. Does the teacher include 'portfolio' types of measures to demonstrate student mastery of specific skills through the use of multiple sources? An example of this might include gauging the "appropriate use of the semicolon" as demonstrated by homework submissions in geography, literature, and history over a one month period, etc.)
g. Does the teacher collaborate with special education staff, counseling, school nursing, and parents, when needed?

The Resource and Special Education Classrooms and Staff:

a. Is there enough staff to effectively work with all the students? What is the student-to-teacher ratio?
b. What is the appropriateness of "fit" for this student, in terms of the needs of the other students in the class? How does the student view the environment? (This would include the teacher, the other students, and the class location, etc.)
c. To what degree are students being *instructed and*/or *assisted* with school work? Is there evidence of 'busy work' or other activities that are not intrinsic to grade level curriculum, or to the goals/objectives stated in the educational plan?
d. How are students with fine motor weaknesses being assisted or accommodated for? Are they provided options for using assistive technology?
e. Is there an avoidance of placing *all students with any disabling condition* into this one class? (Or, for example, is a student with cerebral palsy with movement difficulties, (but doing grade level work for his age,) automatically placed with students with both physical and intellectual impairments, because this is the only class that serves students with special needs?)
f. Similarly, is there avoidance for the placement of any and all students with social, emotional, or other psychiatric conditions into the same class? (For example, are students with severe behavioral problems or conduct disorders put in the same class with, for example, a student with PANS, who may be suffering from sensory overwhelm, social anxiety, and fearfulness?)
g. Does the teacher seem to have the situation 'in hand,' or does she appear overwhelmed and under-assisted?
h. Are materials organized? Do students know where to go to retrieve materials?
i. Is the atmosphere positive to work in? Is there natural lighting for those who may be sensitive to fluorescent lighting, and are there areas where students can concentrate on work without being distracted (such as study carrels, etc.)?
j. Are the walls absent of visual 'clutter' that may be over-stimulating and distracting for some students?

Considerations Regarding Placement into a Residential School, or Segregated School for Students with Special Needs:

a. Is there strong collaboration and agreement among the parents, medical providers, and staff, that this is the most appropriate placement?
b. Have parents or guardians visited the facility?
c. Subjectively and 'qualitatively'[10] speaking, are staff members *nice, kind,* and *respectful* to students and to one other? Is the atmosphere welcoming and receptive?
d. Does staff demonstrate an understanding of the PANS etiology, and do they articulate or make reference to the ways in which PANS can affect the student's schoolwork? Do they make references to how PANS can affect students differently from other students with special learning needs?
e. Is it clear to all parties (including the student to the extent appropriate) what the *goals are* in this placement? Is it understood by all parties that this is not a permanent placement, but a placement that is needed for the shortest amount of time, as indicated by the student's welfare and educational needs? What is the timeline of the placement, and how will this timeline be monitored and adjusted as needed?
f. Is it clear that staff and administration distinguish between unexpected or atypical behaviors resulting from PANS, and similar behaviors resulting from other factors? (If so, how? Is this acknowledged anywhere in the educational plan?)

g. How will the staff's understanding of PANS etiology and related symptoms influence their use of 'disciplinary' techniques?
h. What are the needs of the other students in the school?
i. Is there an extremely low or (preferably) ***no*** incidence of violence among students in the facility?
j. Are the staff trained, certificated, and 'seasoned' in education and special education?
k. Has the student had a chance to visit the facility? Is there anything there that holds promise or hope for him or her there? For example, are there horses or other animals that might be viewed as comforting? Are there any subjects, teachers, technology, teaching style, other students, *anything*- that are seen as 'positives' for the student?
l. Does this placement meet the criteria for *'least restrictive environment'* for that student?
m. If the student suffers from bedwetting, social anxiety, and fear of separation from a parent, how will this be addressed in respectful and supportive ways?
n. What provisions are there for the use of technology?
o. Does the school offer the same-grade curriculum as that offered in non-residential or special schools in that jurisdiction? Do they offer classes for those who are gifted and talented?
p. Is there evidence that the school will provide meals that are in compliance with the dietary needs of the student (such as gluten-free, allergen free, etc.)?
q. Regarding any neuropsychiatric medications that the student may be taking, are staff members aware of potential side effects of these medications? Do they know symptoms to look out for? How are potential side-effects monitored and documented?
r. What is the school's policy regarding travel and accompaniment for hospital and doctors' visits?
s. What is the school's policy regarding unscheduled visits by parents?
t. Does the school have all of the services and support staff that their regular education school counterparts would have (such as speech and occupational therapists, etc.?
u. Does the school offer opportunities for sports and extracurricular activities?

Considerations Regarding Home/Hospital Instruction:

a. Does the team offer a rationale for the amount of instructional time offered at home or in the hospital?
b. Is the teacher certificated and trained in the subject matter being taught? If special education is needed, is the home/ hospital teacher trained and credentialed in that area too?
c. Does this teacher collaborate with the regular and/or special education teacher at the school on a regular basis?

Considerations Regarding Private Schools and Colleges:

a. Does the school clearly disclose their parameters of services for students with special needs (on their web site, literature, school manual, etc.?)
b. Does the school present clear procedures and understandable instructions for obtaining these services?
c. If the school receives federal funding (that makes them subject to Section 504), are related accommodations, modifications, and other services implemented? How is this demonstrated and monitored?
d. If the school is one of a cluster, or system, of private schools (such as those under the auspices of a Catholic diocese, for example), is there a clear policy regarding the parameters of support and

instruction that will be available to students with special needs *from the administration overseeing that cluster of schools*? How is this demonstrated? Are there efforts made by the administration to assure that *all schools* within their purview are providing similar quality of instruction in this area, and have similar levels of support?

e. Does the school seek out assistance and collaboration from the local public school districts when needed?
f. Similar to that in public schools, is there a *team approach* (that can include outside supports) before, and when, difficulties arise?
g. If the school literature states that they accept and support students who have a verified disabling condition, is there faculty at the school *who can competently oversee* that these accommodations and modifications are being put in place?
h. What avenues are there for the parents (or the public) to obtain statistics regarding the percentage of the student body with identified disabilities, including a breakdown of those with medical conditions (OHI) and Specific Learning Disabilities (SLD)? (Is the percentage of students with disabling conditions amongst *overall attendees* similar to that of *the graduating class?)*
i. Are there opportunities for instructors, parents, and the public to address concerns regarding the education of students with special needs? (This not only includes concerns over a particular student, but the quality, type, and direction of services for students with special needs as a group.)
j. Are parents and staff perceived as welcomed participants at school advisory panels, school boards, etc.?
k. In the event that the student is not able to achieve 'as hoped for' at this school, do staff members first assure that any agreed-upon accommodations, etc., have actually taken place? How? Is there *a team approach* (including teachers, parents, outside professionals, the student when appropriate, etc.) implemented when a student is at risk of being *"dismissed"* from this school for poor achievement? Or conversely, is there a sense that decisions have been made "behind closed doors," with little transparency, or recourse, for the family, the student, or teachers?)
l. Finally, if the student *does* qualify for accommodations and modifications because of a verified disabling condition, but *has not received these* at the school (for whatever reason), how do his grades and transcripts take this into account? In other words, if the student eventually transfers to another school, is there any acknowledgement (in transcripts or other accompanying documentation) that grades were based on coursework and tests where needed accommodations *were not provided?* [11]

The Integral Role of District and Governmental Educational Agencies

District and governmental agencies play an integral role in the delivery of educational services to all students, but especially for those with special needs, and even more so when students have medical conditions that warrant the kind of attention that PANS does. At these 'macro' levels of education, support can make the difference between students having access to services, *or not*. This may be even truer for small, rural, or private schools.

Given this need, what might be helpful considerations, as these larger agencies strive to support the schools and students within their purview? Following are a few recommendations.

a. <u>Provide Resources about PANS</u> and its educational implications for teachers and other staff members, which can be assessed by the web.
b. <u>Provide Presentations, Workshops, and Comprehensive Training</u> when needed by a School Nurse or 'outside' provider.

c. Ensure that School Nurses within the Related Jurisdiction(s) are aware of this illness, and are aware of how it may present differently from non-PANS related OCD and other psychiatric disorders.

d. Create Targeted Training (as it relates to a particular student) for educators and other school affiliated providers as needed.

e. Provide Avenues for Advocacy for the student and the family. This may include mediation of disputes regarding educational plans, but can also include 'ombudspersons' who are easily accessible, and who can be spoken to in confidence about concerns and questions regarding the educational process and related care.[12] It may also include questions and concerns about accessing resources with their governance.

f. Provide Information and Access to Resources in the Community that are at cost, no cost, and low cost that can serve these students and families.

g. Provide Opportunities For Parents and Community Members to Collaborate. These include collaboration on advisory boards related to special education, mental health, and public health. They also can include oversight committees to ensure that there is attention and awareness given to PANS and its educational implications. Other points of collaborations would include "Child Find" types of agencies that are expected to seek out, identify, and address potential disabilities in the school aged population.

h. Provide Opportunities For Outreach and Training in The Community Regarding PANS. The following agencies should especially become familiar with the medical and behavioral manifestations of this serious illness. They should also be cognizant of appropriate and effective care and emergency response to individuals affected by PANS-related symptoms.

- Medical Emergency Services
- Police and Law Enforcement
- Fire Departments
- Social Services
- Mental Health Care Agencies
- Juvenile Justice Systems
- Public Health Departments
- Hospitals and Urgent Care Clinics
- Private Schools and Colleges
- Religious Organizations
- Other Non-Profit Organizations that Serve Youth and Young Adults

i. And Last, but Certainly Not Least, Provide Opportunities for Collaboration on PANS-Related Research.

Close collaboration with schools and the communities they represent is needed to provide further research into PANS. This is needed, not only in the fields of medicine and psychiatry, but also in Education, Special Education, Psychology, Social Work, Public Health, Nursing, Ophthalmology and Binocular Vision, and other related areas touched by this illness. There is, of course, a need to continue such *quantitative* studies, whereby, statistics, for example, can evaluate PANS-related behaviors with evidence of virus or bacteria, etc. At the same time, there is also a need for *qualitative* studies too, whereby salient information can be gleaned from interviews and other sources to provide new themes and generate new theory. At all levels, including the master and doctoral levels, such research is needed to obtain more feedback and insight from the parents, siblings, and especially, the PANS-affected students themselves. For it is only through these perspectives, that we can truly come to a more complete understanding of how this formidable illness both manifests, and heals.

Final Thoughts

In closing, if PANS stands alone in its unique, diagnostic hallmark of profound and deleterious effects on behavior and cognitive abilities, so it also stands alone, *thankfully,* in its equally stunning potential for healing and recovery. It is the fragile academic limbo that connects these two disparate states that schools are charged to address. Educators, and the systems that support their work, are sought out for help by desperate loved ones surviving in a world of dysfunction and chaos; where the child, and perhaps even the parents, may have already lost sight of the calm, vibrant, and thriving landscape ahead. Those entrusted to ensure this student's safe academic passage as he transitions from illness to wellness will determine the nature and extent of its educational repercussions. With the expertise, vision, and the conviction of doing what is appropriate and right for this student, a good teacher, in collaboration with the family, and aided by the support of others at the school and larger community, will have the steady hand necessary to help navigate secure passage to the other side, where the student will, once again, sustain himself.

Notes

---

[1] Even through the advent of technology, whereby parents, living in the most remote of areas, can type in key words associated with PANS or PANDAS, and come up with information about the illness on their computers.
[2] This underscores the need for the educational team to be aware of the underlying difficulties that require intervention.
[3] This is, by no means, an exhaustive list, but a sampling of positive indicators.
[4] This will include custodians, kitchen staff and reception staff.
[5] In the US, for example, do they demonstrate compliance with all applicable federal and state laws, regulations, and guidance such as 504, and IDEA?
[6] In other words, is there a staff member who clarifies what the potential **scope** of investigation and services are for the student? (Or, do staff members, or the team facilitator, constrict or limit the discussion to what is already evident?)
[7] Such as those related to results on fine motor, visual processing, and memory skills, etc?
[8] (In the US, and in other countries that similarly recognize these educational rights.)
[9] Perhaps stemming from problems in fine motor skills, memory, organizational factors, etc.
[10] But not ***'just...'***
[11] Thereby rendering such measurements of skills and competencies of questionable reliability and use.
[12] It is important to remember that special education will be new to most of these parents and students. Most will not even be familiar with the *parameters* of what types of services or interventions that are available. Given this limited understanding, they may have no idea then, what is actually in their reach or prerogative to expect or to discuss.

(An) Epilogue

... But Mary Treasured Up All These Things,
And Pondered Them in Her Heart.
- Luke 2:19[1]

I suppose that every mother carries images in her heart of a beloved son's journey through childhood. Chapter portraits- reflecting not so much sequences of time, but of that resonance forged by raw and uncensored emotion, maternal love, and an ethereal perspective held in balance by a reasoning that reason knows not of.[2,3]

I replay even now those darkest of reels, moving portraits seared of desperation and fear, where a numbed panic can extend life-deciding seconds of ordinary time into netherworlds of timeless limbos. But of course, there are no clocks, in any case, in that turbulent confluence of depth, darkness, and silence, where parents must descend to save their drowning child.

In those early years of no diagnosis and misdiagnosis, the desperate attempts to stop our son's descent had led only to myriads of labyrinths, within, well- myriads of labyrinths.[4] *The money, the time, and most preciously, our son's own rapidly-eclipsing boyhood, had been gobbled up by appointments with medical providers who invariably could not heal him.*

How, for all of our sakes, I longed for those fantasized images of the increasingly elusive 'ordinary childhood day.' *Seeking solace through the compassionate confessionals of a few precious others, I would allow myself the inescapable surges of mourning that would ebb and flow along with the illness itself; of grievings for the many childhood memories that my son would never know, his sister would never share, and his father and I would never cherish.*

And yet...

There would mercifully remain an invisible collection of treasured vignettes, pulled out and pondered at will, that would sustain me through it all; signposts that somewhere in my son's body, mind, and spirit, life prevailed.

Indeed, these visual affirmations became my Proofs of Life. *Proof that his body was doing everything in its power to help right itself, but also, Proof, through treasured glimmerings of character, spirit, intelligences, empathy, creativity, resilience, and compassion, that despite everything, my son was choosing to live and to grow- using whatever tools life would still offer him.*

I knew that I was one of the lucky ones.[5] *Over time, the darkest of memories would become gently offset by poignant and powerful ones, not only of my son's steadfast pursuit of life, but also of the kindness, goodness, wisdom, and helpfulness of others. Most especially, I became so grateful to those who, even in the depths of his illness, not only continued to recognize, acknowledge, and appeal to my son's* authentic self, *but also recognize his unique gifts too.*

I suppose it was the treasured images of our son's years in Boy Scouts that extended that golden thread of hope and promise that his capacity for life would invariably triumph.

Before Diana Pohlman would reach out to this unknown, desperate mother in that critical 11th hour of her son's descent;

Before Nurse Practitioner Amy Fishman Smith, in her medical knowledge, wisdom, experience, and astute clinical perception, became the first practitioner (this, following a long parade of pediatricians, psychologists, neurologists, pediatric psychiatrists, developmental psychologists, etc.) to recognize what all of those formerly disregarded symptoms actually were- the glaring indications of a serious, yet treatable *medical condition;*

And before Amy Fishman Smith and Dr. Sunjya Schweig would offer a path back to wellness through antibiotics, intravenous immunoglobulin (IVIG), and other restorative measures;

There was Boy Scouts, and a boy who wanted to be part of it all, and a community that not only accepted him, but saw his potential- even in the depths of this illness, and even before this young man could see it in himself.

One poignantly memorable summer camp would also mark our son's final descent into PANS as well. He would not be back at camp the next year- too exhausted, although paradoxically, already at a turning point in his recovery. It was on that first day of camp, as he nervously embraced this last retreat into wooded wonderland, *that I would be gifted with an especially treasured memory. It would be one that I would take out and ponder at will in the months and years to come. The most bittersweet of scenes, it would be melded of fear, overwhelm, kindness, thoughtfulness, generosity, wisdom, empowerment, risk, and resilience- all rolled into one...*

He is standing on a deck, awaiting his turn for the annual swim test that will allow him to swim in the camp's lake. His troop is one of the first troops to attempt the test that afternoon, leading all of the other groups of boys who stand behind them, waiting excitedly for their turns. I know that he has the ability to swim, so I am not expecting any problems. However, as I stand under the shade of a dark pine tree some distance away, I see him repeatedly ready himself for the plunge, only to then, suddenly stop himself. He keeps looking out at the water and back, at times risking a dip of his toe in the cold mountain water before quickly stepping back to safety on the pier. One by one, as if in lock-step, the other boys jump in and take their turns. I continue to watch my son... and hope. But soon, my eyes become drawn to this unknown swim counselor too. Reminiscent of a great magician, he acts, powerfully, by not taking any action at all. For in no perceptible way does he ever acknowledge my son's overwhelming fear and hesitation, nor the possibility that he may not even be able to do the task at hand. Instead, he nonchalantly allows him to remain on that deck, as the other boys- actually, as all of the other boys in all of the other troops- take their turns. They go on to pass or not pass, but at least they jump in and try. Time passes. It is now nearing sunset, and with everyone else back at their camp sites, I remain encased in the newly found arms of a hollowed redwood, too entranced by this unfolding spectacle to look away; too fearful of swaying fate's hand by even *moving.*

They are now two alone on the deck. The swim counselor could tell him to come back another day, and my son would leave... But he doesn't. From what I can see, he doesn't say much of anything at all, but steadily busies himself with note taking or some other non-essential task that will keep him on deck with my son. *"Who will leave first...?"* I wonder. One minute agonizingly turns into twenty more, and then, in the quiet calm of twilight, I hear a splash. I see his head come up first, instantly followed by extended arms that quickly propel him forward, and I see the counselor smiling as he signals to his unseen partner on the other shore, that a scout is *"on his way to complete the test!"* ... And he does.

Even then, it would be another year before it was confirmed that our son did have what we would later term as PANS, after all. His symptoms of anxiety, obsessive compulsive disorder, and loss of energy, were indeed tied to an autoimmune condition, and to one that was actually treatable.

More than four years since this formal diagnosis, our son still does not talk about PANS much. Perhaps he has not had the distance he needs from it yet, to realize how much this devastating condition has impacted his youth. Nevertheless, there would be untold times when I would take out those treasured images like the one on the deck that day, where, with the empowerment of an unknown, yet benevolent Wizard-Disguised-as-Swim-Counselor, *our son would literally just take that plunge into the unknown, and* 'just do it.'

And this would ultimately portray how he'd choose to carry himself throughout his PANS illness, and throughout his youth (which for too long were intertwined). Despite the brain inflammation affecting his mood, attention, perception, organizational skills, and stamina, he would choose to move forward, in whatever ways he could.

He made up classes when he fell behind academically. He volunteered in his capacity as a Boy Scout, even though he knew that the car rides to volunteer sites would be difficult. He sought out a third Eagle Scout project after the first two he had investigated and planned for fell through. And late one spring night, after an acquaintance became intoxicated and later abandoned by 'friends,' he would stand by and ferry the young person to safety, never mentioning the matter to curious others. And even through the worst of the illness, he would remain sensitive and caring to animals and to those in need. And these actions, in turn, became my treasured images of hope, my Proofs of Life *that I would continue to ponder in my heart.*

And so it happened, that with the support and intervention of others, our son made the transition from illness and dysfunction *to* wellness and function. *Healers, his aunts and uncles, grandparents, sister, precious friends, team mates, coaches, teachers and administrators, and Boy Scout Leaders; all of these people and more, would make this possible.*

This epilogue is about a young man's triumph over a debilitating illness and the adversity that surrounds it. PANS can be a dreadful condition by any measure. At times, it can manifest in such jagged and stunning regression, that it can rock one's notion of what a family is even capable of. In the bleakest of times, it can even question one's notion of what is reasonable or fair in life.

How remarkable is it, then, that this same jagged and stunning phenomena, could somehow result in such positive *trajectories too? Such unexpected trajectories, that by all that is considered* logical, *appear to be just as equivalently* illogical, *in how they can* somehow *wend their way to such positive 'endpoints'?*

...Where, for example, a student who barely 'got by' in school for so many years, would nevertheless find himself doing very well on college entrance exams down the road; or, where a once-winded jogger, who was barely able to walk *to the finishing line*[6] *of the* Midway Run Fundraiser, *would go on to win* first prize *in this same city-wide race four short years later; or, incredibly, that that same weary walker, with perseverance, and with the mentorship of devoted and caring coaches, would find himself all alone, but never more befriended and supported, as the only one in his entire high school that year to qualify for the* California State Finals in Cross Country Running...

Which brings us to our close. It was not that long ago, that anyone (save his Grandpa, of course) would assume that our son would one day have the strength, much less the wherewithal, to envision, reach for, and ultimately attain for his very own, the highest rank within Boy Scouts- that of Eagle Scout. *However, as PANS so blatantly instructs us, life does not always bow to expected trajectories. Of course, as in the healing of PANS, nothing materializes from the efforts and dreams of one person alone. Metamorphoses as striking as these can only be built on scaffolds of collaboration, fueled by wisdom, caring, and truth.*

And these, along with other virtues so exquisitely brought to life by my son's actions and those of others, comprise images of treasured memories that I will continue to ponder in my heart, no matter where our son's journey leads us.

Notes

[1] Taken from The New Testament, (New International Version*)* Retrieved 7/27/15 at http://biblehub.com/luke/2-19.htm

[2] "Le coeur a ses raisons que le raison ne connaît point." Merci à Mr. Blaise Pascal, *Pensées (1670)*

[3] Fortunately, as awareness of PANS continues to expand, and appropriate treatment becomes more immediate, increasing numbers of families will be spared the heart-breaking experience of seeing their child suffer the tremendous fluctuations in dysfunction and behavior as our family did; this while we desperately tried to seek out a correct diagnosis.

[4] Think M.C. Escher here.

[5] Although these pages do not hold enough space to delve into the topic adequately, I know that my greatest fortune in this journey with PANS was to have in my husband, a life partner who stood by us in the fight to save our child.

[6] Finishing, just a hair, before an elderly citizen with a cane.

Resources

Glossary of Common Terms and Acronyms

51/50 (California)
A "51/50" concerns the involuntary confinement of someone who is suspected to have a mental disorder that makes him or her a danger to self, a danger to others, and/or gravely disabled. Section 51/50 of the California Welfare and Institutions Code allows a qualified officer or clinician to involuntarily confine a person for up to 72 hours, during which time he or she is evaluated. Of course, legislation and protocols surrounding the community response to such a crisis will certainly vary- from state to state, and country to country. Factors to the type of response received will depend not only on funding and access to appropriate care, but also on cultural and logistical expectations and beliefs surrounding such crises.

(Section) 504 of the **Rehabilitation Act of 1973** (US)
Section 504 is legislation that guarantees certain rights to people with disabilities, including *fair and reasonable access* to publicly funded programs, including educational programs, and also private schools that receive public funding. Section 504 is widely recognized as the first civil-rights statute for persons with disabilities in the US.

504 Plan (US)
A 504 Plan is a legal document that falls under the provisions of the Rehabilitation Act of 1973. It is designed to plan a program of instructional services to assist students with special needs who do not require Special Education under the guidelines of IDEA.

Adaptive Behavior (US) IDEA
The ability to function effectively and independently in different settings (such as at home, in the community, in new environments, and at school). Such skills typically include communication and social skills (such as using the telephone), daily living skills (such as the use of public transportation, and personal care skills (such as dressing and grooming). A key element in determining degree of adaptive behavior ability is that a student's skills must be compared with others his age.

ADHD
Attention Deficit Hyperactivity Disorder

ADR
Alternative Dispute Resolution. An ADR and mediation are voluntary methods of resolving disputes about educational services that are viewed as being less adversarial than a due process hearing. Requests for obtaining this type of resolution can be made in addition to requests for a due process hearing.

Advocacy
For educational purposes, advocacy concerns the procurement of help in getting services for oneself or one's minor child. It is broadly used to include both paid and unpaid individuals who will speak on behalf of the student, or in any other way, support the student in receiving services and interventions. This can include advice to parents given over the phone regarding rights, or accompaniment of a parent or student to educational meetings, etc.

AT (Assistive Technology)
AT not only refers to computers, but software, walkers, prosthetics, communication boards or any device that helps facilitate particular functions and abilities. *Adapted* technology refers to those devices that are used to increase capabilities in individuals with disabilities.
(*Assessing for Adaptive Technology Needs, Disability Training Network, July 2007 Powerpoint by* Tracey Forman, Texas A&M University; Retrieved 7/05/2015.)

Autism (US) IDEA
(1)(i) "*A* developmental disability significantly affecting verbal and nonverbal communication and social interaction, generally evident before age three, that adversely affects a child's educational performance. Other characteristics often associated with autism are engagement in repetitive activities and stereotyped movements, resistance to environmental change or change in daily routines, and unusual responses to sensory experiences.
(ii) Autism does not apply if a child's educational performance is adversely affected primarily because the child has an emotional disturbance, as defined in paragraph (c)(4) of this section.
(iii) A child who manifests the characteristics of autism after age three could be identified as having autism if the criteria in paragraph (c)(1)(i) of this section are satisfied."
(Source: *Ed.gov. Regulations: Part 300 / A / 300.8*)

Basal Ganglia
The anatomic area of the brain that is most implicated in PANS. Located deep in the upper third area of the brain referred to as the **forebrain** area, the basal ganglia's relay function allows for strong, efficient interconnectedness among different areas of the brain.

CAPD Central Auditory Processing Disorder
(Also known as *Auditory Processing Disorder- APD*), CAPD is used to denote a variety of disorders that affect the way the brain processes auditory information, whereby individuals are able to hear normally, but are not able to process the sounds they hear in the same way as others do. This, in turn, leads to difficulties in recognizing and interpreting these sounds, especially those that compose speech.

CFR
Code of Federal Regulations

Disability- Child with a Disability §300.8) (US) IDEA:
"(a) *General.* (1) Child with a disability means a child evaluated in accordance with §§300.304 through 300.311 as having an intellectual disability, a hearing impairment (including deafness), a speech or language impairment, a visual impairment (including blindness), a serious emotional disturbance (referred to in this part as "emotional disturbance"), an orthopedic impairment, autism, traumatic brain injury, any *other health impairment* [emphasis added], a specific learning disability, deaf-blindness, or multiple disabilities, and who, by reason thereof, needs special education and related services.
(2)(i) Subject to paragraph (a)(2)(ii) of this section, if it is determined, through an appropriate evaluation under §§300.304 through 300.311, that a child has one of the disabilities identified in paragraph (a)(1) of this section, *but only needs a related service* and not special education, the *child is not a child with a disability* under this part.
(ii) If, consistent with §300.39(a)(2), *the related service* required by the child *is considered special education* rather than a related service under State standards, the child would be determined to be a *child with a disability* under paragraph (a)(1) of this section.
(b) Children aged three through nine experiencing developmental delays."
(Source: *Ed.gov. Regulations: Part 300 / A / 300.8*)

Developmental Delay: (US) IDEA
"A child with a disability for children aged three through nine (or any subset of that age range, including ages three through five), may, subject to the conditions described in §300.111(b), include a child—
(1) Who is experiencing developmental delays, as defined by the State and as measured by appropriate diagnostic instruments and procedures, in one or more of the following areas: physical development, cognitive development, communication development, social or emotional development, or adaptive development; and (2) Who, by reason thereof, needs special education and related services."
(Source: *Ed.gov. Regulations: Part 300 / A / 300.8*)

Emotional Disturbance (US) IDEA
"... A condition exhibiting one or more of the following characteristics over a long period of time and to a marked degree that adversely affects a child's educational performance:
(A) An inability to learn that cannot be explained by intellectual, *sensory*, or *health factors* [emphasis added].
(B) An inability to build or maintain satisfactory interpersonal relationships with peers and teachers.
(C) Inappropriate types of behavior or feelings under normal circumstances.
(D) A general pervasive mood of unhappiness or depression.
(E) A tendency to develop physical symptoms or fears associated with personal or school problems.
(ii) Emotional disturbance includes schizophrenia. The term does not apply to children who are socially maladjusted, unless it is determined that they have an emotional disturbance under paragraph (c)(4)(i) of this section.
(Source: *Ed.gov. Regulations: Part 300 / A / 300.8*)

Encopresis
Involuntary soiling of underwear with stool by youth past the age of toilet training.

Enuresis
Having to do with bed-wetting or the release of urine at inappropriate times.

Home/ Hospital Instruction (US)
The provision for school districts to provide (at no cost to the family) instruction to qualified students (who are usually ill or recuperating) at home or in the hospital when these students are not able to attend school.

IDEA (US)
"The Individuals with Disabilities Education Act (IDEA) is a law ensuring services to children with disabilities throughout the nation. IDEA governs how states and public agencies provide early intervention, special education and related services to more than 6.5 million eligible infants, toddlers, children and youth with disabilities." US Dept of Education- Building the Legacy: IDEA 2004
(http://idea.ed.gov/)

IEE (US) IDEA
Under IDEA, the student has the right to obtain an *Independent Educational Evaluation* (outside of the school district of the student's residence).

IEP Goals (US) IDEA
Goals developed annually by the IEP team to address the student's identified needs. As stated in the IEP document, these goals describe what the child is expected to do, or learn, within a 12-month period.

IEP Objectives (US) IDEA
Short term bench marks to quantify, or measure, progress towards a goal. For example, with a goal being, "Hans will increase social communication skills as measured by the benchmarks listed below:", an objective might be, "By June of 20__, Hans will engage in conversational turn-taking with others across 3-4 conversational turns, 4/5 opportunities to do so (with topics initiated by self or others), as observed and documented by teacher and paraprofessional."

IEP Team (US) IDEA
Participants who are involved in the IEP Process and that, at a minimum, include parents, teachers, administrators, the student (if appropriate), and evaluators.

(IFSP) Individualized Family Service Plan
Similar to an IEP, but applies primarily to infants or toddlers with disabilities. In this case, the family is considered the recipient of services. The IFSP must include all medical and health services that a student requires, even if provision of one or more of these service falls outside of the school district's obligations (IDEA law; Sec. 303.344(e)).

IHSP/IHP/IHCP Individualized Health Services Plan/Individual Health Plan/Individual Health Care Plan/School Nursing Plan, etc.
A written plan that outlines the safe delivery of health services by a school or school district to the student. Students whose health status requires professional nursing observation or intervention, administration of procedures, or the use of a health device need an IHSP *(Taken from American Academy of Pediatrics, 2015)*

Immunoglobulins
Immunoglobulins are proteins that help make up antibodies. There are five types, or classes of immunoglobulins: IgG, IgA, IgM, IgD and IgE. Whereas some Immunoglobulins can reach adult levels by puberty (like IgG), others like IgA (associated with the secretory system), typically take longer to develop (into the teen years).

Individualized Education Program (IEP)
A written document that describes the educational plan for a student with a disability.

Intellectual Disability (US) IDEA
(Formally referred to as Mental Retardation) Referring to "significantly subaverage general intellectual functioning, existing concurrently with deficits in adaptive behavior and manifested during the developmental period, that adversely affects a child's educational performance."
(Source: *Ed.gov. Regulations: Part 300 / A / 300.8*)

IVIg
Intravenous Immunoglobulin is the transfer of (pooled) donor immunoglobulin, specifically containing IgG antibodies, into the body intravenously. It is usually given when less invasive treatments, such as the use of antibiotics, are not sufficient.

LD/SLD Specific Learning Disability (US) IDEA
A disorder in one or more of the basic psychological processes involved in understanding or in using language, spoken or written, that may manifest itself in the imperfect ability to listen, think, speak, read, write, spell, or to do mathematical calculations, including conditions such as perceptual disabilities, brain injury, minimal brain dysfunction, dyslexia, and developmental aphasia... does not include learning problems that are primarily the result of visual, hearing, or motor disabilities, of (intellectual disability), of emotional disturbance, or of environmental, cultural, or economic disadvantage.
(Source: *Ed.gov. Regulations: Part 300 / A / 300.8*)

(LRE) Least Restrictive Environment (US) IDEA
LRE concerns the education of students with disabilities in regular classes (with appropriate aids and supports whenever possible) *before* transferring them to a more restrictive (or separate) learning environment. IDEA requires that states have in procedures in place that, "to the maximum extent appropriate, children with disabilities, including children in public or private institutions or other care facilities, are educated with children who are not disabled, and that special classes, separate schooling, or other removal of children with disabilities from the regular educational environment occurs only when the nature or severity of the disability is such that education in regular classes with the use of supplementary aids and services cannot be achieved satisfactorily." (20 USC 1412(5)(B).)

Manifestation Determination IEP (US) IDEA
Meetings set up to determine whether or not a student's violation of behavior is a direct result of the student's disability. If the IEP team *determines that the violation was caused by the student's disability* [emphasis added], he or she cannot be expelled. At the same time, if a student possesses, uses or sells drugs on campus or brings a weapon to school, they can be expelled regardless of their disability. Expelled students in this case often attend school. Remember that being expelled means that the child has been removed from the school district. It does not mean that the child no longer attends school. Usually, students who have been expelled receive their education at an alternative site provided by the County Department of Education.

Mental Retardation (US) IDEA (See ***Intellectual Disability***)

Molecular Mimicry
"Structural, functional or immunological similarities shared between macromolecules found on infectious pathogens and in host tissues. Molecular mimicry plays an important role in immune responses to infection and in autoimmune diseases. Infection may induce autoimmune responses which attack and destroy body tissues or organs. Normally, the body is tolerant to self-antigens which are present in individual tissues. In autoimmune disease, tolerance is abrogated to self-antigens, and tissues or organs are destroyed by the immune system. Molecular mimicry of a self-antigen by an infectious pathogen, such as bacteria and viruses, may trigger autoimmune disease due to a cross reactive immune response against the infection. Cross-reactive antigen–antibody and T cell–antigen reactions are used to identify the mimicking macromolecules on the pathogen and in tissues or organs. These parameters define the concept of molecular mimicry." (Taken from Cunningham, 2009).
Molecular Mimicry is said to occur when structural, functional, or immunological similarities shared between macromolecules are found on *both* infectious pathogens (such as Strep or Lyme) *and* an individual's own body tissues. In vulnerable individuals, such similarities are recognized to trigger a 'misdirected' autoimmune response, whereby *both* the foreign pathogen and the individual's own body tissues or organs, are attacked and destroyed by that individual's own immune system.

MOU Memorandum of Understanding
An MOU usually refers to an agreement between school districts and outside agencies to provide services. For example, a school district might contract with an outside agency, such as the County Health department, to obtain the services of a nurse for a student.

Multiple Disabilities (US) IDEA
Two or more impairments that occur at the same time (such as intellectual disability and blindness, or 'medically fragile' and orthopedic impairment), "the combination of which causes such severe educational needs that they cannot be accommodated in special education programs solely for one of the impairments. Multiple disabilities do not include deaf-blindness."
(Source: *Ed.gov. Regulations: Part 300 / A / 300.8*)

Münchausen Syndrome by Proxy (**MSBP** or **MBP**)
This is a behavior pattern in which a care provider makes up, exaggerates, or induces mental or physical health problems in those who are in their care.

Neurotransmitters
Neurotransmitters are brain chemicals that communicate information throughout the brain and body. Neurotransmitters are responsible for relaying signals between neurons (nerve cells), and they help to facilitate a number of bodily functions, including the regulation of appetite, sleep, and energy levels. They also play an important role in regulating mood and thought processes, and are involved in our ability to focus and remember things.

OAH (US)
Office of Administrative Hearings. This office deals with disputes/due process surrounding a student's rights to a fair and appropriate education.

Other Health Impairment (OHI) (US) IDEA
Of special significance for students who are affected by PANS, OHI concerns "having limited strength, vitality or alertness, including a heightened alertness to environmental stimuli, that results in limited alertness with respect to the educational environment, that—(i) Is due to chronic or acute health problems such as asthma, attention deficit disorder or attention deficit hyperactivity disorder, diabetes, epilepsy, a heart condition, hemophilia, lead poisoning,

leukemia, nephritis, rheumatic fever, and sickle cell anemia; and (ii) Adversely affects a child's educational performance."
(Source: *Ed.gov. Regulations: Part 300 / A / 300.8*)

Orthopedic Impairment (US) IDEA
A severe orthopedic impairment that adversely affects a child's educational performance. The term includes impairments caused by a congenital anomaly, impairments caused by disease (e.g., poliomyelitis, bone tuberculosis), and impairments from other causes (e.g., cerebral palsy, amputations, and fractures or burns that cause contractures). (Source: *Ed.gov. Regulations: Part 300 / A / 300.8*)

PANDAS
Pediatric Autoimmune Neuropsychiatric Disorder Associated with Streptococcal Infections.

PANS
Pediatric Acute-onset Neuropsychiatric Syndrome.

PITANDS
Pediatric Infection Triggered Autoimmune Neuropsychiatric Disorders.

PL 94-142 (US)
Public Law 94-142, also called the *Education for All Handicapped Children Act,* was legislated to assure that "all children with disabilities have available to them ... a free appropriate public education which emphasizes special education and related services designed to meet their unique needs."
(Source: *Ed.gov. Regulations: Part 300 / A / 300.1)*
It is thought of as one of the initial acts of legislation that recognized the need for, and implementation of, Special Education in the United States.

Plasmapheresis
Plasmapheresis is the removal, treatment, and return of (components of) blood plasma from blood circulation.

Primary Disabling Condition (US) IDEA
The main condition that warrants educational intervention. It is usually, that condition that warrants the most concern, or is the most pervasive or debilitating for the student. Sometimes students are said to have multiple disabilities, such as blindness and orthopedic impairments.

Procedural Safeguards (US) IDEA
Procedural Safeguards Includes the right to "participate in all meetings, examine all educational records, and obtain an independent evaluation of the child. Parents have the right to written notice when the school proposes to change or refuses to change the identification, evaluation or placement of a child. The law includes several ways to resolve disputes including mediation, a "Resolution Session" and due process hearings. Procedural safeguards include legally binding written mediation agreements and confidentiality"
(http://www.wrightslaw.com)

Putamen
Structure of the brain that is a part of the basal ganglia; often implicated in PANS.

Related Services
Services to help a child with a disability benefit from special education, (such as Speech therapy to help with communication or mobility training to help with transportation).

Special Education (US) IDEA
"Special education is specially designed instruction, at no cost to the parents, to meet the unique needs of a child with a disability." This includes " instruction conducted in the classroom, in the home, in hospitals and institutions, and in other settings; ... (It includes) instruction in physical education and special education, (2) *Special education* includes each of the following, if the services otherwise meet the requirements of paragraph (a)(1) of this section—(i) Speech-language pathology services, or any other related service, if the service is considered special education rather than a related service under State standards;(ii) Travel training; and (iii) Vocational education."
(Source: ***Ed.gov***. *Regulations: Part 300 / A / 300.8*)

Speech or Language Impairment (US) IDEA
Refers to "a communication disorder, such as stuttering, impaired articulation, a language impairment, or a voice impairment, that adversely affects a child's educational performance."
(Source: *Ed.gov. Regulations: Part 300 / A / 300.8*)

Supplementary Aids and Services (US) IDEA
Determined by the IEP team and are intended to improve student access to learning and participation in academic, extracurricular, and nonacademic activities and settings. The IEP team must determine what supplementary aids and services a child will need, and specify them in the IEP.

TBI Traumatic Brain Injury (US) IDEA
"An acquired injury to the brain caused by an external physical force, resulting in total or partial functional disability or psychosocial impairment, or both, that adversely affects a child's educational performance. Traumatic brain injury applies to open or closed head injuries resulting in impairments in one or more areas, such as cognition; language; memory; attention; reasoning; abstract thinking; judgment; problem-solving; sensory, perceptual, and motor abilities; psychosocial behavior; physical functions; information processing; and speech. Traumatic brain injury does not apply to brain injuries that are congenital or degenerative, or to brain injuries induced by birth trauma." (Source: *Ed.gov. Regulations: Part 300 / A / 300.8*)

UDL Universal Design for Learning
"A set of principles for curriculum development that give all individuals equal opportunities to learn. UDL provides a blueprint for creating instructional goals, methods, materials, and assessments that work for everyone--not a single, one-size-fits-all solution but rather flexible approaches that can be customized and adjusted for individual needs" (National Center on Universal Design for Learning, 2014).

USC (US)
United States Code (or in this case, laws affecting student rights to a fair and appropriate education).

Visual Impairment (including Blindness) (US) IDEA
"Impairment in vision that, even with correction, adversely affects a child's educational performance. The term includes both partial sight and blindness." (Source: *Ed.gov. Regulations: Part 300 / A / 300.8*)

References

American Academy of Pediatrics National Guidelines Regarding Individualized health services plans (2015) http://www.nationalguidelines.org

American Cancer Society Cancer Facts and Figures, 2014 (Retrieved April 1, 2005) http://www.cancer.org/research/cancerfactsstatistics/cancerfactsfigures2014/

The American Medical Association Home Medical Encyclopedia: An A-Z Reference Guide to over 5000 Medical Terms (Vol. I and II (1989) Clayman, C B (Ed.) Random House NY.

American Printing House for the Blind (2014) "Annual Report 2014: Distribution of Eligible Students Based on the Federal Quota Census of January 7, 2013 (Fiscal Year 2014)." Accessed July 28, 2014, from http://www.aph.org/federal-quota/dist14.html.

American Psychiatric Association. (2013). Diagnostic and Statistical Manual of Mental Disorders (5th Ed.). Arlington, VA: American Psychiatric Publishing.

Ayres, A. J. (2005). Sensory integration and the child: understanding hidden sensory challenges (25th anniversary ed., rev. and updated / by Pediatric Therapy Network Los Angeles, CA: WPS.

Bear, M. F., Connors, B. W. & Paradiso, M. A. (2001) Neuroscience: Exploring the Brain, Second Edition, Lippincott Williams & Wilkins, pp 473-482.

Ben-Pazi, H., Stoner., J. A., & Cunningham, M. W. (2013). Dopamine Receptor Autoantibodies Correlate with Symptoms in Sydenham's Chorea. *PLoS ONE*,*8*(9), e73516. doi:10.1371/journal.pone.0073516.

Ben-Sasson, A., Carter, A. S., & Briggs-Gowan, M. J. (2010) The development of sensory over-responsivity from infancy to elementary school Journal of Abnormal Psychology.

Ben-Sasson, A., Carter, A. S.,& Briggs-Gowan, M. J. (2009) Sensory over-responsivity in elementary school: prevalence and social-emotional correlates Journal of Abnormal Psychology.

Benedek, T. G. (2006). The History of Bacteriologic Concepts of Rheumatic Fever and Rheumatoid Arthritis. Semin Arthritis Rheum 36:109-123.

Bernstein, G. A., Victor, A. M., Pipal, A. J., & Williams, K. A. (2010) Comparison of clinical characteristics of pediatric autoimmune neuropsychiatric disorders associated with streptococcal infections and childhood obsessive-compulsive disorder. J Child Adolesc Psychopharmacol. Aug; 20(4):333-40.

Booth, J. R., Wood, L., Lu, D., Houk, J. C., & Bitan, T. (2007) Brain Research. The role of the basal ganglia and cerebellum in language processing. Feb 16; 1133(1):136-44. Epub 2006 Dec 26.

Brimberg, L., Benhar, I., Mascaro-Blanco, A., Alvarez, K., Lotan, D., Winter, C., Klein, J., Moses, A. E., Somnier, F. E., Leckman, J. F., Swedo, S. E., Cunningham, M. W., & Joel, D. (2012) Behavioral, Pharmacological, and Immunological Abnormalities after Streptococcal Exposure: A Novel Rat Model of Sydenham Chorea and Related Neuropsychiatric Disorders. Neuropsychopharmacology. Aug; 37(9):2076-87. doi: 10.1038/npp.2012.56. Epub 2012 Apr 25.

Candelaria Greene, J. F. (2015) Unpublished survey of family members, providers, and survivors of PANS regarding PANS and Education (2013-2015), collected as UC Berkeley Visiting Researcher Scholar, Berkeley, California.

Chakravarthy, V. S., Joseph, D., & Bapi, R. S. (2010) What do the basal ganglia do? A modeling perspective. Biol Cybern Sep;103(3):237-53. doi: 10.1007/s00422-010-0401-y. Epub 2010 Jul 20.

Chang, K., Frankovich, J., Cooperstock, M., Cunningham, M., Latimer, M. E., Murphy, T. K., Pasternack, M., Thienemann, M., Williams, K., Walter, J., Swedo, S. E. & from the PANS Collaborative Consortium. (2015) Clinical Evaluation of Youth with Pediatric

Acute-Onset Neuropsychiatric Syndrome (PANS): Recommendations from the 2013 PANS Consensus Conference Journal of Child and Adolescent Psychopharmacology. February 2015, 25(1): 3-13. doi:10.1089/cap.2014.0084.

Chen, J. Y., Wang, E. A., Cepeda, C., & Levine, M. S. (2013) Dopamine imbalance in Huntington's disease: a mechanism for the lack of behavioral flexibility. Front Neurosci. 2013 Jul 4;7:114. doi: 10.3389/fnins.2013.00114. eCollection 2013.

Columbia University Medical Center (CUMC) Newsroom: How Recurrent Strep A Infections Affect the Brain: Newly discovered route by which immune cells reach the brain may underlie an autoimmune neuropsychiatric disorder in children. (2015) http://newsroom.cumc.columbia.edu/blog/2015/12/15/strepabrain/

Corbett, B., Schupp, C., Levine, S., & Mendoza, S. (2009). Comparing Cortisol, Stress, and Sensory Sensitivity in Children with Autism. Autism Research, 2, 39-49.

Cox, C. J., Sharma, M., Leckman, J. F., Zuccolo, J., Zuccolo, A., Kovoor, Swedo, S .E., Cunningham, M. W. (2013). Brain Human Monoclonal Autoantibody from Sydenham Chorea Targets Dopaminergic Neurons in Transgenic Mice and Signals Dopamine D2 Receptor: Implications in Human Disease. *Journal of Immunology (Baltimore, Md. : 1950)*, *191*(11), 10.4049/jimmunol.1102592. doi:10.4049/jimmunol.1102592.

Craig, G. (2011). The EFT Manual. Energy Psychology Press, Santa Rosa, CA.

Cunningham, M. W. (2000) Pathogenesis of Group A Streptococcal Infections. Clinical Microbiology Reviews, Vol. 13, No. 3, 2000, pp. 470-511. doi:10.1128/CMR.13.3.470-511.

Cunningham, M. & Perry, H. (2008) Autoimmunity and behavior: Sydenham's chorea and related disorders. Paper presented at the 9th International Congress of Neuroimmunology; Fort Worth, TX. 2008.

Cunningham, M. W. (2009) Molecular Mimicry; Published Online: 15 SEP 2009 DOI: 10.1002/9780470015902.a0000958.pub2 2001 John Wiley & Sons, Ltd.

Cunningham, M. W. (2014) Rheumatic fever, autoimmunity, and molecular mimicry: the streptococcal connection. Int Rev Immunol. 2014 Jul-Aug; 33(4):314-29. doi: 10.3109/08830185.2014.917411. Epub 2014 Jun 3.

Davies, P. L. & Gavin, W. J. (2007) Validating the diagnosis of sensory processing disorders using EEG technology *American Journal of Occupational Therapy 61, 176-189.*

deBettencourt, L. U. Difference between 504 Plan and IDEA: From the Council for Exceptional Children (retrieved 2/2015) http://school.familyeducation.com/special-education/ada/38439.html.

Delazer, M., Domahs, F., Lochy, A., Karner, E., Benke, T., Poewe, W. (2003) Number processing and basal ganglia dysfunction: a single case study Neuropsychologia Volume 42, Issue 8, 2004, pp 1050–1062.

Dooley, P., Wilczenski, F. L., & Torem, C. (2001). Using an activity schedule to smooth school transitions. Journal of Positive Behavior Interventions, 3, 57-61.

Dunn, W., Smith, B. M., & Ors. (2002). Sensory-process issues associated with Asperger Syndrome. American Journal of Occupational Therapy, 56, 97-102.

English, P. C. (1991) Emergence of rheumatic fever in the nineteenth century. In: Rosenberg C, Golden J, eds. Framing disease: studies in cultural history. New Brunswick, NJ: Rutgers University Press, 1991:20–32.

Federal Register regulations-to-implement the equal employment provisions of the Americans with Disabilities Act https://www.federalregister.gov/articles/2011/03/25/2011-6056/

Findlay, J. M. & Gilchrist, I. D. (2003) Active vision: The psychology of looking and seeing. Oxford; New York: Oxford University Press, Series: Oxford psychology series, no. 37.

REFERENCES

Frankovich, J., Thienemann, M., Pearlstein, J., Crable, A., Brown, K., & Chang, K. (2015) Multidisciplinary clinic dedicated to treating youth with pediatric acute-onset neuropsychiatric syndrome: Presenting characteristics of the first 47 consecutive patients. J Child Adolesc Psychopharmacol. 2015 Feb;25(1):38-47. doi: 10.1089/cap.2014.0081.

Frick, S. M., & Hacker, C. (2009). Listening with the whole body. Madison: Vital Links.

Hall, L., & Case-Smith, J. (2007). The effect of sound-based intervention on children with sensory processing disorders and visual-motor delays. The American Journal of Occupational Therapy , 61, 209-215.

Hasbi, A., O'Dowd, B. F., George, S. R. (2011) Dopamine D1-D2 receptor heteromer signaling pathway in the brain: emerging physiological relevance. Mol Brain 4: 26.

Heller, S., (2002) Too Loud, Too Bright, Too Fast, Too Tight. New York: Harper Collins.

Hergüner, S., Kilinçaslan, A., Görker, I., & Tüzün, U. (2007) Serotonin-selective reuptake inhibitor-induced enuresis in three pediatric cases. J Child Adolesc Psychopharmacol. Jun;17(3):367-9.

Herrero, M. T., Barcia, C.,& Navarro, J. M. (2002) Functional anatomy of thalamus and basal ganglia. Childs Nerv Syst. Aug; 18(8):386-404. Epub 2002 Jul 26.

Hikosaka, O. (1989) Role of basal ganglia in saccades. Rev Neurol (Paris). 145(8-9):580-6.

Hirschtritt, M. E., Hammond, C. J., Luckenbaugh, D., Buhle, J., Thurm, A. E., Casey, B. J., & Swedo, S. E. (2009) Executive and attention functioning among children in the PANDAS subgroup) Child Neuropsychol. Mar;15(2):179-94. Epub 2008 Jul 11.

Hong, C., Press, L. J., & Visual Factors in Childhood Behavioral Disorders (Retrieved 7/15 at http://www.visionhelp.com/visual-factors-in-childhood-behavioral-disorders/ and http://www.pressvision.com/pdf/hong_press.pdf

Howard, P. (2000) The Owner's Manual for the Brain: Everyday applications from mind-brain research, 2nd edition. Austin, TX: Bard Press.

Ings, S. (2008). A natural history of seeing: The art and science of vision. pp 17-18, 44-47 Publisher: New York: W.W. Norton.

Johnson, D. R., Kurlan, R., Leckman, J., Kaplan, E.L. (2010) The human immune response to streptococcal extracellular antigens: clinical, diagnostic, and potential pathogenetic implications. Clin Infect Dis. 2010 Feb 15;50(4):481-90. doi: 10.1086/650167.

Kabat-Zinn, J. (1996) Full Catastrophe Living (Revised Edition): Using the Wisdom of Your Body and Mind to Face Stress, Pain, and Illness. London: Piatkus.

Kirvan, C.A., Swedo, S.E., Heuser, J.S., Cunningham, M.W., (2003) Mimicry and Auto-antibody mediated neuronal Signaling Cells in Sydenham Chorea, Nature Medicine 9, 914 - 920 (2003) http://www.pandasnet....NMpaper[1].pdf.

Kirvan, C. A., Swedo, S. E., Snider, L. A., & Cunningham, M. W. (2006) Antibody-mediated neuronal cell signaling in behavior and movement disorders. J Neuroimmunol 179: 173–179 *Epub* 2006.

Kirvan, C. A., Swedo, S. E., Kurahara, D., & Cunningham, M. W. (2006) Streptococcal mimicry and antibody-mediated cell signaling in the pathogenesis of Sydenham's chorea. Autoimmunity. 39(1):21-9. http://www.pandasnet...NICaMKinase.pdf.

Kirvan, C. A., Cox, C. J., Swedo, S. E., & Cunningham, M. W. (2007) Tubulin is a neuronal target of autoantibodies in Sydenham's chorea. J Immunol. Jun 1;178(11):7412-21.

Kovacevic, M., Grant, P., & Swedo, S. E. (2015) Journal of Child and Adolescent Psychopharmacology. February 2015, 25(1): 65-69. doi:10.1089/cap.2014.0067.

Kumar, A., Williams, M., Muzik, O. & Chugani, H. (2014) Basal ganglia inflammation in children with neuropsychiatric symptoms J Nucl Med. 2014; 55 (Supplement 1):306.

Larson, K., Russ, S., Kahn, R. S., & Halfon, N. (2007) Patterns of Comorbidity, Functioning, and Service Use for US Children with ADHD. Pediatrics.

Latimer, M. E., L'Etoile, N., Seidlitz, J., & Swedo, S. E. (2015) J Child Adolesc Psychopharmacol. Therapeutic plasma apheresis as a treatment for 35 severely ill children and adolescents with pediatric autoimmune neuropsychiatric disorders associated with streptococcal infections.Feb;25(1):70-5. doi: 10.1089/cap.2014.0080. Epub 2015 Feb 6.

Leckman, J. F., King, R. A., Gilbert, D. L., Coffey, B. J., & Singer, H. S., et al. (2011) Streptococcal upper respiratory tract infections and exacerbations of tic and obsessive-compulsive symptoms: a prospective longitudinal study. J Am Acad Child Adolesc Psychiatry 50: 108–118 e103.

Lehrman, S. (2008) *Nurture into Nature Meet Your New Brain*) Cal Alumni Magazine Volume 119(2) March/April.)

Leisman, G., Melillo, R. & the PANDAS Resource Network. (2013) A Comprehensive Analysis of Research on the Diagnoses and Treatment for Pediatric Automimmune Neuropsychiatric Disorder (PANDAS/PANS).

Lewin, A. B., Storch, E. A., Mutch, P. J., & Murphy, T. K. (2011) Neurocognitive functioning in youth with pediatric autoimmune neuropsychiatric disorders associated with streptococcus. J Neuropsychiatry Clin Neurosci. 2011 Fall;23(4):391-8. doi: 10.1176/appi.neuropsych. 23.4.391.

Martino, D., Tanner, A., Defazio, G., Church, A. J., Bhatia, K. P., Giovannoni, G., & Dale, R. C. (2005) Tracing Sydenham's chorea: historical documents from a British paediatric hospital. Arch Dis Child. May; 90(5):507-11.

McDermott, N. (2008) New online database reveals touching tales of the first Great Ormond Street patients: http://www.dailymail.co.uk/news/article-1101696/New-online-database-reveals-touching-tales-Great-Ormond-Street-patients.html#ixzz3Uc15P5pX (retrieved, March 2015).

Morgan, M. (2005). The Midbrain (Gray Matter). Chelsea House Publications, Philadelphia.

Moretti, G., Pasquini, M., Mandarelli, G., Tarsitani, L., & Biondi, M. (2008). What every psychiatrist should know about PANDAS: a review. Clin Pract Epidemol Ment Health 4: 13. http://www.ncbi.nlm....5-0179-4-13.pdf.

Murphy, M. L., & Pichichero, M. E. (2002). Prospective identification and treatment of children with pediatric autoimmune neuropsychiatric disorder associated with group A streptococcal infection (PANDAS) Arch Pediatr Adolesc Med. 2002;156(4):356–61. [PubMed].

Murphy, T. K., Storch, E. A.,& Strawser, M. S. (2006). Selective serotonin reuptake inhibitor-induce behavioral activation in the PANDAS subtype, Primary Psychiatry, 2006;13(8):87-89, http://mbldownloads....06PP_Murphy.pdf.

Murphy, T. K., Kurlan, R., & Leckman, J. (2010). The immunobiology of Tourette's disorder, pediatric autoimmune neuropsychiatric disorders associated with Streptococcus, and related disorders: a way forward. *J Child Adolesc Psychopharmacol* 20 (4): 317–31.

Murphy, T. K., Storch, E. A., Turner, A., Reid, J. M., Tan, J., & Lewin, A. B. (2012). Clinical Factors Associated with PANDAS J Pediatr Feb; 160(2): 314–319.

Murphy, T. K., Patel, P. D., McGuire, J. F., Kennel, A., Mutch, P. J., Parker-Athill, E. C., Hanks, C. E., Lewin, A. B., Storch, E. A., Toufexi, M. D., Dadlani, G. H., & Rodriguez, C .A. (2015). Characterization of the Pediatric Acute-Onset Neuropsychiatric Syndrome Phenotype Journal of Child and Adolescent Psychopharmacology. February 2015, 25(1): 14-25. doi:10.1089/cap.2014.0062.

National Diabetes Statistics Report, 2014 www.diabetes.org National Federation for the Blind https://nfb.org/blindness-statistics Retrieved April, 2015.

Nelson, K., & Bruner, J. S. (2006). Narratives from the Crib. Cambridge, Mass: Harvard University Press.

REFERENCES

Pavone, P., Bianchini, R., Parano, E., Incorpora, G., Rizzo, R., Mazzone, L., & Trafiletti, R.R. (2004) Anti-brain antibodies in PANDAS versus uncomplicated streptococcal infection. Pediatr Neurol 2004, 30:107-10.

Pederson, R.A. and Troost, B.T. (1981) Stroke Abnormalities of Gaze in Cerebrovascular Disease in Current Concepts of Cerebrovascular Disease. Stroke, Vol 12, No 2, 1981.

Perlmutter, S. J., Leitman, S. F., Garvey, M. A., Hamburger, S., Feldman, E., Leonard, H. L., & Swedo, S. E. (1999): Therapeutic plasma exchange and intravenous immunoglobulin for obsessive-compulsive disorder and tic disorders in childhood. Lancet 1999, 354:1153-1158.

Poynton, F. J., & Paine, A. (1900) The etiology of rheumatic fever. Lancet 1900;2:1306-7.

Poynton, F. J., & Paine, A. (1900)The etiology of rheumatic fever. Lancet 1900;2:861-9, 932-5.

Poynton, F. J., & Paine, A. (1901) Some further investigations upon rheumatic fever. Lancet 1901;1260-5, 1261.

Puget Sound ESD (2010) Office of Special Services, A Parent & Educator Guide to Free Appropriate Public Education. March, 2010.

Purves, D., Augustine, G. J., Fitzpatrick, D., et al., editors.(2001) Neuroscience. 2nd edition. Sunderland (MA): Sinauer Associates. Projections from the Basal Ganglia to Other Brain Regions. Available from: http://www.ncbi.nlm.nih.gov/books/NBK10860/.

Ram, G., & Chinen, J. (2011) Infections and immunodeficiency in Down syndrome. Clinical and Experimental Immunology. 2011;164(1):9-16. doi:10.1111/j.1365-2249.2011.04335.x.)

Reynolds, S., & Lane, S. (2009). Sensory Overresponsivity and anxiety in children with ADHD. American Journal of Occupational Therapy, 63, 433-440.

Robinson, R. (2008) New Roles for the Basal Ganglia in Learning and Memory Neurology Today 17 July 2008; Volume 8(14); p 24.

Rosenberg, C., & Golden, J., (eds). Framing disease: studies in cultural history. New Brunswick, NJ: Rutgers University Press, 1991:20–32.

Saadati, H., Babri, S., Ahmadiasl, N., & Mashhadi, M. Effects of Exercise on Memory Consolidation and Retrieval of Passive Avoidance Learning in Young Male Rats. Asian J Sports Med. 2010 Sep;1(3):137-42.

Sansosti, F .J., Powell-Smith, K. A., & Kincaid, D. (2004). A research synthesis of social story interventions for children with autism spectrum disorders. Focus on Autism and Other Developmental Disabilities, 19, 194-204.

Santa Barbara Community College (Retrieved 2/15) High School vs. College Regulations related to disability and accommodations http://www.sbcc.edu/dsps/*policiesprocedures/.*

Segen's Medical Dictionary (2011). Retrieved March 20 2015 from http://medical-Dictionary.thefreedictionary.com/autoimmune+response.

Siegel, D. J. (2007) The Mindful Brain: Reflection and Attunement in the Cultivation of Well-Being, New York: W.W. Norton.

Siegel, D. J. & Bryson, T. P. (2014) No Drama Discipline The Whole-Brain Way to Calm the Chaos and Nurture Your Child's Developing Mind. New York: Bantam.

Singer, H. S., Gilbert, D. L., Wolf, D. S., Mink, J. W., & Kurlan, R. (2012) Moving from PANDAS to CANS.J Pediatr. 2012 May;160(5):725-31. doi: 10.1016/j.jpeds.2011.11.040. Epub 2011 Dec 22.

Snider, L. A., & Swedo, S. E. (2004) PANDAS: Current Status and Directions for Research. Mol Psychiatry. Oct;9(10):900-7.

Snider, L. A., Lougee, L., Slattery, M., Grant, P.,& Swedo, S. E. (2005) Antibiotic prophylaxis with azithromycin or penicillin for childhood-onset neuropsychiatric disorders. Biol Psychiatry. 57(7):788-92.

South Carolina Department of Education, Office of Nutrition Programs Frequently Asked Questions About IHP's http://ed.sc.gov/agency/se/Instructional-Practices-and- evaluations/documents/FAQ_About_IHPs_Aug2013final. pdf August 8, 2013.

Starr, M. S., & Rayner, K. (2001) Eye movements during reading: some current controversies TRENDS in Cognitive Sciences Vol.5 No.4 April 2001.

Steele, M. M., & Steele, J. W. (2003) Teaching Algebra to Students with Learning Disabilities. Mathematics Teacher, 96(9) Dec 2003.

Storch, E. A. Murphy, T. K., Geffken, G. R., Mann, G., Adkins, J., Merlo, L. .J., Duke, D., Munson, M., Swaine, Z., & Goodman, W. K. (2006) Cognitive-behavioral therapy for PANDAS-related obsessive-compulsive disorder: findings from a preliminary waitlist controlled open trial. J Am Acad Child Adolesc Psychiatry. 2006 Oct;45(10):1171-8.

Swedo, S.E., Leonard, H.L., Schapiro, M.B., Casey, B.J., Mannheim, G.B., Lenane, M.C., Rettew, D.C. (1993) Sydenham's chorea: physical and psychological symptoms of St Vitus dance. Pediatrics. Apr;91(4):706-13.

Swedo, S.E. (1994) Sydenham's Chorea: A Model for Childhood Autoimmune Neuropsychiatric Disorders *JAMA.* 1994;272(22):1788-1791. doi:10.1001/jama.1994.03520220082035.

Swedo, S. E., Leonard, H. L., Mittleman, B. B., Allen, A. J., Rapoport, J. L., Dow, S. P., Kanter, M. E., Chapman, F., & Zabriskie, J. (1997) Identification of Children With Pediatric Autoimmune Neuropsychiatric Disorders Associated With Streptococcal Infections by a Marker Associated With Rheumatic Fever", Am J Psychiatry 154:1, January 1997 http://ajp.psychiatr...t/154/1/110.pdf.

Swedo, S. E., Leonard, H. L., Garvey, M., Mittleman, B., Allen, A. J., Perlmutter, S.,Lougee, L., Dow, S., Zamkoff, J., & Dubbert, B. K. (1998) PANDAS: Clinical Description of the First 50 Cases; Am J Psychiatry. Feb;155(2):264-71.

Swedo, S. E. (2002). Pediatric autoimmune neuropsychiatric disorders associated with streptococcal infections (PANDAS) Mol Psychiatry. 7 Suppl 2 (s2): S24–5. doi:10.1038/sj.mp.4001170. PMID 12142939. http://www.nature.com/mp/journal/v7/n2s/pdf/4001170a.pdf.

Swedo, S. E., Leonard, H. L., & Rapoport, J. L. (2004) The pediatric autoimmune neuropsychiatric disorders associated with streptococcal infection (PANDAS) subgroup: separating fact from fiction. Pediatrics:113(4):90711 http://pediatrics.aa...print/113/4/907.

Swedo, S. E., & Grant, P. J. (2005): Annotation: PANDAS: a model for human autoimmune disease. J Child Psychol Psychiatry 46:227-234.

Swedo, S. E., Leckman, J. F., & Rose. N. R. (2012) From Research Subgroup to Clinical Syndrome Modifying the PANDAS Criteria to Describe PANS (Pediatric Acute-onset Neuropsychiatric Syndrome) Pediatrics and Therapeutics 2:113.

Swedo, S. E., Seidlitz, J., Kovacevic, M., Latimer, M. E., Hommer, R., Lougee, L.,& Grant, L. P. (2015) Clinical presentation of pediatric autoimmune neuropsychiatric disorders associated with streptococcal infections in research and community settings. Journal of Child and Adolescent Psychopharmacology. February 25(1): 26-30.

Sweeney, M. S. (2009) Brain: The Complete Mind: How it Develops, how it Works, and how to Keep it Sharp. National Geographic Books, Washington, DC.

Tanner, A. (2008) Small and special: a website of the origins of the Great Ormond Street Hospital for Children, Presentation given (GOSH) at HARG General meeting January 2008 retrieved at http://www.healtharchives.org/HARGpapers.html March 2015.

REFERENCES

Taranta, A., & Stollerman, .G. H. (1956) The relationship of Sydenham's chorea to infection with group A streptococci. The American Journal of Medicine , Volume 20 , Issue 2 , 170 - 175.

Thamotharampillai, D., Smith, D., Knowland, D., Hsu, M., Platt, M., Bittner-Eddy, P., Cohen, B., Southern, P., Latimer, E., Harley, E., Dritan Agalliu, D., & Cleary, P. P.. (2016) Group A Streptococcus intranasal infection promotes CNS infiltration by streptococcal-specific Th17 cells. J Clin Invest. 2016;126(1):303-317.

Tomchek, S., & Dunn, W. (2007). Sensory processing in children with and without autism: A comparative study using the short sensory profile. The American Journal of Occupational Therapy, 61, 190-200.

Tona, J., & Posner, T. (2011) PANDAS/PITAND Recognizing and treating children with Pediatric Autoimmune Neuropsychiatric Disorders in OT From: nysota information on PANDAS-PITAND and OT.

Tsushima, M., Tsushima, W., Tsushima, V., Lim, N., Madrigal, E., Jackson, C., & Mendler, M. H. (2013).Use of ImPACT to diagnose minimal hepatic encephalopathy: an accurate, practical, user-friendly internet-based neuropsychological test battery. Dig Dis Sci. 2013 Sep;58(9):2673-81. doi: 10.1007/s10620-013-2668-z. Epub 2013 Apr 27.

U.S. Department of Education Office for Civil Rights (2011) Students with Disabilities Preparing for Postsecondary Education: Rights and Responsibilities: http://www2.ed.gov/about/offices/list/ocr/transition.html.

Williams, R. C. Jr. (1983). Rheumatic fever and the streptococcus. Another look at molecular mimicry. Am J Med. 75(5):727-730.

Wolosin, S. M., Richardson, M. E., Hennessey, J. G., Denckla, M. B., & Mostofsky, S. H. (2009). Abnormal Cerebral Cortex Structure in Children with ADHD. Hum Brain Mapp. 30(1):175-184.

Woodcock, R. W., McGrew K. S., & Mather N. (2001) Woodcock-Johnson III. Itaska, IL: Riverside Publishing.

Yaddanapudi K., Hornig M., Serge R., De Miranda J, Baghban, A., Villar, G., & Lipkin, W. I. (2010). Passive transfer of streptococcus-induced antibodies reproduces behavioral disturbances in a mouse model of pediatric autoimmune neuropsychiatric disorders associated with streptococcal infection. Mol Psychiatry. 15(7):712-726.

Websites and Other Resources

Education and Learning Aides

Pandasnetwork.org http://pandasnetwork.org/
ACN Latitudes on Line. http://latitudes.org/
National Dissemination Center for Children with Disabilities: http://nichcy.org
Tourette Syndrome Association; tsa-usa.org
CHADD sites (ADHD/ Executive Function) www.chadd.org
The American Occupational Association; http://www.aota.org/
Intervention Central- Academic Resources for Accommodations, Study Skills, RTI: http://www.interventioncentral.org/--
Association of Educational Therapy *http://*www.aetonline.org/
Anxiety Disorders Association of America: http://www.adaa.org/living-with-anxiety/children/childhood-anxiety-disorders
Child Anxiety (Consumer-oriented Child Anxiety web site: http://www.childanxiety.net National Resource Center on ADHD: www.help4adhd.org --
School Psychology Resources for Psychologists, Parents and Educators: http://www.schoolpsychology.net/
Learning Disabilities Association of America: http://www.ldanatl.org
NLDA, Nonverbal Learning Disorders Association http://www.nlda.org/ NLDline http://www.nldline.com/
Handwriting without Tears www.hwtears.com
Sensory Integration - American Occupational Therapy Association http://www.aota.org/practice/children-youth/si.aspx
Universal Design for Learning www.udlcenter.org
Khan Academy - (Best for pre-college and college age). www.khanacademy.org
ADDitude Support for students with ADHD and Learning Disabilities thttp://www.additudemag.com/adhd/article/824.html
https://www.overdrive.com/ (Borrow eBooks, audiobooks, and more from your local public library - All you need is a library card.

Safeguarding Student Rights and Advocacy

The Office of Civil Rights Section 504
www.ed.gov/ocr; http://www2.ed.gov/about/offices/list/ocr/504faq.htm
Office of Special Services, A Parent & Educator Guide to Free Appropriate Public Education-in-March, 2010
http://www.k12.wa.us/HealthServices/pubdocs/504ManualFinal.pdf
The Office of Civil Rights (504 grievances) How to file a Grievance through 504
http://www.ed.gov/about/offices/list/ocr/complaintintro.html.
Wrights Law advocacy and Special Education Law: Center for Parent Information and Resources http://www.wrightslaw.com;
What You Need to Know About IDEA 2004: http://www.wrightslaw.com/idea/art.htm
10 Tips: How to Use IDEA 2004 to Improve Your Child's Special Education:
http://www.wrightslaw.com/idea/art/10.tips.steedman.htm
Individualized Education Programs (IEPs): http://www.wrightslaw.com/info/iep.index.htm
U.S. Department of Education http.//www.ed.gov/
information/advocacy from Learning Disabilities advocacy (LD on Line) www.ldonline.com
Information on IDEA (2004): http://www.ldonline.org/features/idea2004
(In California) California Department of Education/Special Education, Special Education Local Planning Agency; California Department of Education Sacramento, (916) 445-4613
http://www.cde.ca.gov/index.asp
Implementation of California's Special Education Laws and Regulations
Notice of Procedural Safeguards (US) www.k12.wa.us/SpecialEd/pubdocs/PS.pdf;

Assistive Technology

Learning Ally (formerly RFBD)—Audio books and resources: http://www.learningally.org/
Books Aloud: Audio Library Online: http://www.booksaloud.org/
Book Share-Books and Periodicals for those with disabilities affecting their processing of print: (free to US students with qualifying conditions, and low cost to everyone else.)
http://www.bookshare.org/
Don Johnson software: Skill Development Draft Builder, Co-Writer, Read Out Loud & Write Out Loud:
http://www.donjohnston.com/Dragon Naturally Speaking:
Ginger Online advanced grammar and spell check: http://www.gingersoftware.com/
Inspiration—Brainstorming and outlining software: www.inspiration.com
Kurzweil software: Web-based literacy software: www.kurzweiledu.com/

LiveScribe pen/recorder device: http://www.livescribe.com/
Library of Congress Audio Books http://www.loc.gov/nls/
Reading Naturally-Reading phonics and fluency development: www.readingnaturally.com
Intel Reader device: http://www.intel.com/healthcare/reader/video.htm
The National Federation of the Blind: http://www.nfb.org/nfb/Products_and_Technology.asp?SnID=962155186
Assistive Technology for Students with Disabilities:
Mathletics: http://www.mathletics.com.au/home.asp
Multiple graphic organizers:http://udltechtoolkit.wikispaces.com/Graphic+organizers
Luminosity software: Reclaim your brain: http://www.lumosity.com/

Assistive Technology for Reading:
http://natri.uky.edu/assoc_projects/qiat/documents.html
Assistive Technology Resource Guide (Georgia Project for AT): http://www.gpat.org/resources.aspx?PageReq=GPATConsider
Matrix to evaluate/ select adjustable technology-reviews & summarizes features: http://www.techmatrix.org/Home
Voice Dictation Software: http://shop.nuance.com/store/nuanceus/Content/pbPage.dns-page1

(*Note:* Thanks to *Georgia Project for AT* for additional resources regarding Assistive Technology.)

Health Resources
Online video by Doctors Cleary and Agalliu explaining their findings regarding PANS' mechanism: (https://www.youtube.com/watch?v=HlpzWGS6f60).
IMPACT testing 1(877) 646-7991 impacttest.com
(California) Golden Bear Sleep and Mood Research Clinic ww.ocf.berkeley.edu/~ahsleep/main.html
Univ. of Cal. Binocular Vision Dept. providing evaluation for binocular vision and visual perception (510) 642-2020.
Eye exercise resources www.eyecanlearn.com/
Scales to view symptoms of OCD and Tic (*YGTSS)* severity: https://www.div12.org/assessment-repository/
Meditation and Mindfulness Resources:
Videos on YouTube (Daniel Siegel: Discussing The Science of Mindfulness; Discussing. Empathy and Cognition. Brain Hand Model).
Stop, Think, Breathe: Mindfulness meditations (http://stopbreathethink.org/)
Free Guided Meditations (UCLA) (http://marc.ucla.edu/body.cfm?id-22)
Mindfulness for Teens (CD By Gina Biegel)
Books:
The Mindful Brain: Reflection and Attunement in the Cultivation of Well-Being. Daniel Siegel (W.W. Norton, 2007).
The Mindful Child, Susan Kaiser Greenland (Atna Books, 2010).
Peaceful Piggy Mediation. Kerry Lee MacLean (Albert Whitman and Company, 2004).

Other
Google Scholar, National Center for Complementary and Alternative Medicine (National Institute of Health, NCCAM.NIH.GOV;
Support for Families with Disabilities: http://www.supportforfamilies.org/
Great Schools-: http://www.greatschools.net/content/specialNeeds.page
College Board Services for Students with Disabilities (SSD) (US) https://www.collegeboard.org/students-with-disabilities (609) 771-7137
Documentation for College Board http://www.ets.org/disabilities/documentation/
http://professionals.collegeboard.com/testing/ssd/application/eligible/requirements
Association on Higher Education and Disabilities https://www.ahead.org

APPENDICES

Appendix I. The Yale-NIMH PANS Scale*

This is adapted from the original form, which can be found on pandasnetwork.org. (2016) Used with permission. For downloadable version, see PANDAS Network/Understanding PANS PANDAS Symptoms/ Scales (http://pandasnetwork.org/understandingpandaspans/about-pandaspans/symptoms/).

Date: ______ **Name:** ______ **Gender: F M** ______

Date of birth: ______ **Date of onset:** ______

Informants: ______ **Telephone numbers** ______

Version: June 6, 2012

DOMAIN	One week prior to first onset	Week following first onset	Current (past 7 days)
Date			
Obsessive-compulsive symptoms (0-25) (5 X the worst of the OC symptoms)**			
Associated neuropsychiatric (NP) symptoms (0-25) (sum of the 5 (of 7) worst NP domains)***			
1. Anxiety symptoms (0-5)			
2. Extreme moodiness and/or depression (0-5)			
3. Irritability or aggressive behavior (0-5)			
4. Learning/cognitive symptoms, confusion (0-5)			
5. Behavioral regression (0-5)			
6.A. Sensory symptoms (0-5)			
6.B. Hallucinations (0-5)			
6.C. Motor symptoms (0-5)			
7.A. Urinary symptoms (0-5)			
7.B. Sleep disturbance, fatigue (0-5)			
7.C. Dilated pupils (0-5)			
TOTAL SYMPTOMS (0-50)			
Impairment (0-50)			
TOTAL SCORE (0-100)			

* Provided by co-authors Drs. James Leckman (Yale) and Susan Swedo (NIMH), *unpublished data.* Collaborative acknowledgements to Drs. Paul Grant (NIMH), Kyle Williams, (Massachusetts General Hospital) and Margo Thienemann (Stanford University). With the help of Diana Pohlman, Keith Moore, and many other parents.

**Six Obsessive-compulsive symptoms domains are presented. Rate all of them. However, on the above table only enter the score of the most severe domain (times 5; 0-25).

***Seven Associated symptom domains are presented. Rate all of them. However, for each domain one or more symptom sets are listed. On the above table, only enter the score of the most severe symptom set for each domain (0-5).

THE YALE NIMH PANS SCALE

SYMPTOM SEVERITY RATING SCALE (use these anchor points for each of the symptoms)

Severity *(rate each of the symptoms listed on the following pages for the past week)*	
NONE No evidence of specific symptoms and behaviors	**0**
MINIMAL Specific symptoms and/or behaviors are present but are only evident occasionally and not a major source of difficulty.	**1**
MILD Specific symptoms and/or behaviors are present during the past week, and are episodically a source of some distress and difficulty.	**2**
MODERATE Specific symptoms and/or behaviors are present every day and are a source of distress and difficulty.	**3**
SEVERE Specific symptoms and/or behaviors are present every day and are severe resulting in a great deal of distress and difficulty.	**4**
EXTREME Specific symptoms and/or behaviors are always present and are extremely severe resulting in an extreme degree of distress and difficulty.	**5**

BOC INDICATORS: If multiple time points will be rated on this form, please use the following indicators:
"**B**" = Symptom severity one week ***Before*** the onset of the first episode of illness "**O**" = Symptom severity during the week following the initial ***Onset*** of symptoms "**C**" = ***Current*** symptom severity during the past week

---

Date: __________ **Name:** __________________________ **Informant:** ____________________

I. CORE Obsessive-compulsive Symptoms (circle and rate ALL symptoms that have been present in the past week). Use the "BOC" indicators if multiple time points are being scored (above).

Obsessive-compulsive symptoms **0=Absent 1= Minimal 3=Moderate 4= Severe 5= Extreme**	**0**	**1**	**2**	**3**	**4**	**5**
Intrusive and persistent obsessional worries (anxieties) about dirt and germs and related washing compulsions (circle obsessions and/or compulsions)						
Intrusive and persistent obsessional worries (anxieties) about harm to self or others and related compulsions; a need to tell or confess (this symptom domain may be closely related to separation worries, but rate both if both are present						
Intrusive and persistent obsessional worries (anxieties) about sexual or religious thoughts or behaviors and related rituals and compulsions						
Intrusive obsessional worries about symmetry and related compulsions: ordering, counting, *or* arranging; a need to touch, tap or rub, or a need for things to feel, look, *or* sound 'just right'						
Intrusive and persistent obsessional worries (anxieties) about collecting and hoarding						
Restrictive and/or avoidant food intake symptoms; Eating or feeding disturbance (including but not limited to apparent lack of interest in eating or food; avoidance based on the sensory characteristics of food; or concern about aversive consequences of eating) resulting in a refusal to eat (atypical anorexia) or a marked decrease in food intake						
Miscellaneous. The need to know or remember; Fear of saying certain things; Fear of not saying just the right the right thing; Intrusive (non-violent) images; Intrusive sounds, words, music or numbers; Need to repeat activities (e.g. in/out of a doorway, up/down from chair); The need to involve another person (usually a parent) in ritual (e.g. asking a parent to repeatedly answer the same question; Mental rituals other than checking/counting; Excessive list making: Other						
Severity of all the above Obsessive-compulsive symptoms (over the past week) Five times this rating [0-25] should be entered on p. 1						

Yale-NIMH PANS Scale (continued)

II. ASSOCIATED SYMPTOMS (circle and rate ALL symptoms that have been present inthe past week). Use the "BOC" indicators if multiple time points are being scored.

1. Anxiety Symptoms **0=Absent 1= Minimal 3=Moderate 4= Severe 5= Extreme**	**0**	**1**	**2**	**3**	**4**	**5**
Separation anxiety – need to maintain proximity to person, a familiar location, or a thing						
General anxiety						
Unfounded irrational fears and/or phobias						
Panic episodes						

2. Emotional lability, depression **0=Absent 1= Minimal 3=Moderate 4= Severe 5= Extreme**	**0**	**1**	**2**	**3**	**4**	**5**
Emotional lability – mood swings- moodiness						
Depression with or without suicidal or self injurious thoughts						

3. Increased irritability or aggressive behavior **0=Absent 1= Minimal 3=Moderate 4= Severe 5= Extreme**	**0**	**1**	**2**	**3**	**4**	**5**
Increased irritability; defiant/irrational demands; reactive aggressive behavior; temper tantrums; rage attacks						

4. Behavioral Regression 0=Absent 1= Minimal 3=Moderate 4= Severe 5= Extreme	**0**	**1**	**2**	**3**	**4**	**5**
Behavioral regression ("baby talk," behavior atypical for actual chronological age)						
Change in personality						

5. School performance Concentration/ Learning **0=Absent 1= Minimal 3=Moderate 4= Severe 5= Extreme**	**0**	**1**	**2**	**3**	**4**	**5**
Difficulties in attention, concentration or learning – unable to concentrate or a clear problem with immediate or short term memory						
Loss of academic skills – especially math or in reading or writing						
Confusion						

Yale-NIMH PANS Scale (continued)

6.A. Sensory symptoms 0=Absent 1= Minimal 3=Moderate 4= Severe 5= Extreme	0	1	2	3	4	5
Heightened sensitivity to light, the way things "feel" (tags or labels) or "sound" or other sensory stimuli – such as smell or taste; a need to touch things in a specific way; how things "look" including spatial distortion (eg. objects appear closer than they actually are)						
6.B. Hallucinations 0=Absent 1= Minimal 3=Moderate 4= Severe 5= Extreme	**0**	**1**	**2**	**3**	**4**	**5**
Visual or auditory hallucinations						
Yale-NIMH PANS Scale (continued)						
6.C. Motor symptoms 0=Absent 1= Minimal 3=Moderate 4= Severe 5= Extreme	**0**	**1**	**2**	**3**	**4**	**5**
Dysgraphia (loss of ability to draw, copy figures and/or write letters)						
Motoric hyperactivity and/or adventitious movements - kicking, spitting, flailing, rolling, or stomping (do not rate tics here); unable to stay still						
Piano playing finger movements						
Simple motor tics or vocal tics (grunting, squeaking, etc)						
Complex motor or vocal tics including; spitting, obscene words or actions, repeating words or actions changes in rate or pitch of speech						

7.A. Urinary symptoms 0=Absent 1= Minimal 3=Moderate 4= Severe 5= Extreme	0	1	2	3	4	5
Urinary frequency or increased urge to urinate; daytime or night; inability to						
7.B. Sleep disturbance - Fatigue 0=Absent 1= Minimal 3=Moderate 4= Severe 5= Extreme	**0**	**1**	**2**	**3**	**4**	**5**
Sleep problems (lengthy bedtime rituals, insomnia, inability to sleep; hypersomnia, nightmares)						
Extreme tiredness or fatigue						
7.C. Dilated pupils 0=Absent 1= Minimal 3=Moderate 4= Severe 5= Extreme	**0**	**1**	**2**	**3**	**4**	**5**
Dilated pupils –"terror stricken look"						

Yale-NIMH PANS Scale (continued)

Impairment Rating

Use the "BOC" indicators if multiple time points are being scored (see p. 2).

Name: ____________________

Informant: ____________________

IMPAIRMENT ***(past week)***		
NONE	**0**	
MINIMAL Symptoms associated with subtle difficulties in self-esteem, family life, social acceptance, or school or job functioning (infrequent upset or concernabout tics *vis a vis* the future, periodic, slight increase in family tensions because of symptoms; friends or acquaintances may occasionally notice or comment about symptoms in an upsetting way).	**10**	
MILD Symptoms associated with minor difficulties in self-esteem, family life, social acceptance, or school functioning.	**20**	
MODERATE Symptoms associated with some clear problems in self-esteem family life, social acceptance, or school or job functioning (episodes of dysphoria, periodic distress and upheaval in the family, frequent teasing by peers orepisodic social avoidance, periodic interference in school performance because of PANS symptoms.	**30**	
SEVERE Symptoms associated with major difficulties in self-esteem, family life, social acceptance, or school functioning.	**40**	
EXTREME Symptoms associated with extreme difficulties in self-esteem, family life, social acceptance, or school functioning (severe depression with suicidal ideation, disruption of the family (separation/divorce, residential placement), disruption of social ties - severely restricted life because of social stigma and social avoidance, removal from school).	**50**	

Appendix II: Examples of Symptoms of Obsessions and Compulsions

Taken from the CY-BOCS Checklist**

The CY-BOCS is another important tool that is used to assist in identifying and monitoring parameters of PANS-associated behaviors (presence, type, severity, and frequency) throughout the course of the illness.

Examples from Obsessions Checklist Items marked "*" may or may not be OCD phenomena.

- **Contamination Obsessions** (concern with dirt, germs, certain illnesses (e.g., AIDS), concerns or disgust with bodily waste or secretions (e.g. urine, feces, saliva), *other)*
- **Aggressive Obsessions** (fear of harming self or others, fear of blurting out obscenities or insults, *other)*
- **Sexual Obsessions** (forbidden or perverse sexual thoughts, images, impulses, sexual behavior towards others (aggressive), *other)*
- **Hoarding / Saving Obsessions** (fear of losing things, *other)*
- **Magical Thoughts / Superstitious Obsessions** (lucky / unlucky numbers, colors, words, *other)*
- **Somatic Obsessions** (excessive concern with illness or disease *, excessive concern with body part or aspect of appearance (e.g. dysmorphophobia) *, *other)*
- **Religious Obsessions** (excessive concern or fear of offending religious objects, an excessive concern with right / wrong morally, *other)*
- **Miscellaneous Obsessions** (such as a need to know or remember, the fear of saying certain things, *other)*

Examples from Compulsions Checklist Items marked "*" may/ may not be OCD phenomena.

- **Washing / Cleaning Compulsions** (excessive or ritualized hand washing, excessive cleaning of items, *other)*
- **Checking Compulsions** (checking locks, toys, school books / items, etc., *other)*
- **Repeating Rituals** (rereading, erasing, or rewriting; needing to repeat activities, *other)*
- **Counting Compulsions** (objects, certain numbers, words, etc., *other)*
- **Ordering / Arranging** (the need for symmetry / evening up, etc., *other)*
- **Hoarding / Saving Compulsions** (difficulty throwing things away, saving bits of paper, string, etc., *other)*
- **Excessive Games / Superstitious Behaviors** (touching an object or self-certain number of times as a
- routine game to avoid something bad from happening, *other)*
- **Rituals Involving Other Persons (the need to involve another person (usually a parent) in ritual** (e.g. asking a parent to repeatedly answer the same question, making mother perform certain mealtime rituals involving specific utensils) *, *other)*
- **Miscellaneous Compulsions** (mental rituals other than checking / counting , need to tell, ask or confess, Trichotillomania (hair-pulling), *other)*

** These are only a few of the many examples taken from the Yale-Brown Obsessive-Compulsive Scale (CY-BOCS) for Children.

(Storch EA, Murphy TK, Adkins JW, Lewin AB, Geffken GR, Johns NB, Jann KE, Goodman WK. The children's Yale-Brown obsessive-compulsive scale: psychometric properties of child- and parent-report formats. J Anxiety Disord. 2006;20(8):1055-70. Epub 2006 Feb 28.)

Appendix III: Examples of Motor Tics and Phonic Tics

Taken from the Yale Global Tic Severity Scale (YGTSS) Section B: Tic Severity**

The YGTSS is used as a tool to assist providers and families establish and monitor parameters of PANS-associated behaviors (presence, type, severity, and frequency) throughout the course of the illness.

1. Motor Tics

a. ***Simple Motor Tics:*** (Rapid, Darting, "Meaningless")
Eye blinking, Eye movements, Nose movements, Mouth movements, Facial grimace, Head jerks/movements, Shoulder shrugs, Arm movements, Hand movements, Abdominal tensing, Leg or foot or toe movements, Other

b. ***Complex Motor Tics*** *(Slower, "Purposeful")*
Eye gestures or movements, Mouth movements, Facial movements or expressions, Head gestures or movements, Shoulder gestures, Arm or hand gestures, Writing tics, Dystonic postures, Bending or gyrating, Rotating, Leg or foot or toe movements, Tic-related compulsive behaviors (touching, tapping, grooming, evening-up), Copropraxia, Self-abusive behavior, Paroxysms of tics (displays), Disinhibited behavior*, Other

(The rater is asked to) describe any orchestrated patterns of sequences of motor tic behaviors.

2. Phonic Tics

a. ***Simple Phonic Symptoms:*** (Fast, "Meaningless" Sounds):
Sounds, noises: (circle: coughing, throat clearing, sniffing, grunting, whistling, animal or bird noises), Other

b. ***Complex Phonic Symptoms****:* (Language: Words, Phrases, Statements):
Syllables, Words: Coprolalia, Echolalia, Palalalia, Blocking, Speech atypicalities, Disinhibited speech*

(The rater is asked to) describe any orchestrated patterns or sequences of phonic tic behaviors.

**Denotes an item that is not included in the rating of ordinal scales.*

(**Taken from Leckman, J. F., Riddle, M. A., Hardin, M. T., Ort, S. I., Swartz, K. L., Stevenson, J., & Cohen, D. J. (1989). The Yale Global Tic Severity Scale: initial testing of a clinician-rated scale of tic severity. Journal of the American Academy of Child and Adolescent Psychiatry 28(4), 571. To view complete scale, please refer to local providers, and to online resources such as *https://www.div12.org/assessment-repository/*.)

Appendix IV: Sample Letters to Initiate Services

The following letters include the types of information that are often used in communications to initiate services with schools. *These letters are much longer than what are typically written.* Often, letters are limited to one or two pages, where a brief explanation is given, and more information is presented later on (in person, on the phone, or in accompanying letters from providers). The intent here is meant *only* to provide the reader with possible areas to consider and include.

Moreover, this is only a guide. It is always wise to look at the procedural guidelines and recommendations specific to one's community, district, and governmental agencies, and consider seeking advice from those knowledgeable of the most recent guidelines in one's region as well.

Sample Letter to Provider (Medical, Psychological, Other) to Document the Need for Services
(Example for a modified day with Home/Hospital Instruction)

Family Address or Letterhead
(Date)
Re: Mark J. D. DOB 6/24/09
Medical Record Number: 62496JAC

Dear Dr. C.,

(State specific need and rationale.) We are hoping that you would be willing to help us obtain a shorter, or "modified," school day and "home-hospital instruction" for our son, Mark.[1 2] As you know, he is currently a seventh grader at Meadowlake Middle School here in Mangas Unified School District. (We have included the name of the principal and other contact information on the attached paper.)

Specifically, we are asking for your help because Mark has generally been absent most school days until 11:30, and so is missing a lot of instruction. This has been happening, despite his working with a social worker on bedtime and wake up routines. (We have also put some restrictions on his use of computers and other types of technology in the evening that may interfere with his sleep.)

(Describe behaviors in detail, noting how often they occur and where.) As we mentioned at previous medical appointments with you, we are seeing severe anxiety, symptoms of obsessive compulsive disorder (such as taking a very long time to brush his teeth and disinfect his comb each time he uses it), and tics (where he coughs and hits a wall simultaneously). We typically see this about forty times a day when he is at home. Moreover, he has great difficulty traveling in cars to school because of motion sickness and anxiety. Although he typically complains of headaches and tiredness in the morning, he seems to have good energy levels in the afternoon and evening.

(State school comments and observations, and the student's perspective.) All of the above behaviors and symptoms affect Mark's ability to get to class on time, and as a result, they seriously impact his ability to function and participate at school. We are at a point where Mark is getting F's for the first three classes of the day, simply because he is not there. The teacher stated yesterday that he has the skills to do the work, but at this point, he is just not keeping up. At school, the teachers say that Mark looks preoccupied and that he often is not looking at them when they are talking. However, Mark tells us that he *is* paying attention, but that he just doesn't like to look at them. For all classes that involve writing, reading, or math, the instructors state that he currently needs double the time (his peers need) to take tests and to finish any of his assignments.

(Include what outside therapy you are also doing to help with symptomatology). We are in the process of working with a new therapist familiar with Cognitive Behavioral Therapy and relaxation techniques. However, we have not noticed any changes in his ability to cope or manage his fears or anxiety, as of yet.

(Cite academic and other strengths.) The other academic consideration is that, fortunately, he is doing well in the English class (that he is presently taking on-line). The English teacher says that he is probably doing better with the on-line course because there are no "cooperative learning activities" that require him to interact with other students, and read and write material quickly. The school allowed him to take this course on-line because in our school district, if a student fails a subject, which Mark did last fall, they offer to pay the expense of a course on-line (which he takes after school.) Mark continues to enjoy chess and an occasional game of soccer; although, as we said at our last doctor's appointment, he often runs out of energy while doing any sports or athletic activity.

(Provide a summary with specific recommendations, so that the medical provider can also be specific when she writes the letter on your behalf.) In sum, we hope that you will be able to recommend that Mark receive instruction at home 3 times a week for ninety minutes (each instructional visit for his first three classes of the day (English, History, and Social Studies) and then attend school for the last 3 periods of the day. We also request that you mention that he may be out of school because of medical and other appointments related to his health.

(Include interventions that you know may be inappropriate or ineffective for the student.) To be clear, Mark is <u>unable</u> to take classes on-line *independently,* because of his severe attentional and anxiety symptoms, which are, of course, directly related to his PANS diagnosis. However, he *can manage* the on-line courses, if they are facilitated by an instructor or assistant who is physically with him while he is on- line. (This is especially important for his pre-Algebra course.)

We would be thankful for any help you can give us.

Thanks in advance for your help,

Sincerely,

Mr. and Mrs. D. (555) 333-3333

SAMPLE OF LETTER TO SCHOOL REQUESTING A SCHOOL NURSING PLAN

(For a student who currently does not require special education or a '504.'[3] (US)

Family Address or Letterhead

Date

Dr. Nancy Johnson
Principal/Head master or Superintendent
Mayfair Unified School District
1952 Silver Lake Drive
Minnoton, California 89666

Re: Hans J. D. DOB 6/24/09

Dear Dr. Johnson,

We are writing to you about our son, Hans, who is presently enrolled in Mrs. E. H's fourth grade class at Hinkley Elementary School.

We are requesting that you initiate services through a school nursing plan, (in Mayfair Unified School District referred to as an "IHCP"), as he is currently receiving evaluations and related medical treatment for the autoimmune condition Pediatric Acute-onset Neuropsychiatric Syndrome (PANS).[4]

Specifically, we are asking for this health care plan, so that a registered nurse can facilitate and monitor aspects of his unique nursing needs as it relates to his education. Attached is the contact information from his treating provider, Dr. S., along with her letter that both confirms Hans's diagnosis, and provides related recommendations during his school day.

Our immediate concerns surround instruction time lost from medical appointments, transportation concerns, and needs surrounding the intermittent administration of medications. In addition, we want to ensure that the school becomes aware of the strict dietary constraints that Hans's doctor has advised.

Moreover, we are worried about the increase in his facial tics (also associated with this illness), and are eager to know how we can address this, so that Hans's participation in school activities do not suffer (or worse, that he does not become a target of bullying or harassment). As everyone who has worked with him knows, Hans has always been a kind and caring boy who has gotten along easily with others. We would not want symptoms of this illness to begin to interfere with his social development and interaction with other students.

If you have any questions or need to discuss this further, please call us at (349) 666-1124 or alternatively on my husband Oliver's cell phone (443) 484-2968.

Thanks in advance for your assistance.

Sincerely,

Lisa and Oliver D.

SAMPLE OF LETTER TO SCHOOL REQUESTING A REFERRAL FOR ASSESSMENTS FOR SPECIAL EDUCATION AND 504 (US) [5]

Family Address or Letterhead

Date

Dr. Nancy Johnson
Director of Special Education
Mayfair Unified School District
1952 Silver Lake Drive
Minnoton, California 89666

Re: Hans J. D. DOB 6/24/09

Dear Dr. Johnson,

We are writing to you about our son Hans, who is presently enrolled in Mrs. E. H's fourth grade class at Hinkley Elementary School.

We are concerned because he is not progressing at school, and are hereby requesting that he be assessed to determine eligibility for special education services and support. We believe that he may qualify for an IEP and services under ***Other Health Impaired*** (OHI), as he is currently receiving evaluations and related medical treatments for the autoimmune condition Pediatric Acute-onset Neuropsychiatric Syndrome (PANS).[6]

As part of these assessments, we are anxious to review Hans's health history and his current health and related needs with a registered school nurse within the district. We feel strongly that in order for Hans to fully participate and benefit from his education, he will need the assistance of a school nurse who can implement a nursing plan to assist him as he recovers from this illness. In this regard, we look forward to meeting with her, and would welcome the opportunity for her to interview us at our home. In this way, she can preview his current medications, and observe and discuss other modifications that we have made here at home to help accommodate for his needs.

Regarding his participation at school, we have become aware through his teacher, Mrs. H., that Hans does not seem to be as attentive as he was in the fall. He is forgetful of what he has just heard, and of what he's supposed to do next. He also has difficulty completing his seat work and homework as easily as his classmates. We are seeing similar difficulties at home too.

Moreover, although he has always been an outstanding student in Math (as evidenced by his good report cards and State-wide testing scores) we are noticing that he is now starting to fall behind. His numbers are difficult for him to write, and for others to read. He also has problems with organizing his math columns when he is trying to solve long division and multiplication problems.

We have also spoken to Mrs. H. about Hans's speech. We have all noticed that he seems to carry saliva in his mouth, and that his pronunciation of words is not as understandable as it used to be. Moreover, we have concerns about his understanding of language in general, and notice that he speaks to others less than he used to.

Another area of concern has to do with his cursive handwriting and his drawing ability. Both have become increasingly messy, despite Hans taking a lot of time and effort to do his best. (A simple five sentence homework assignment two nights ago, for example, took Hans forty minutes to complete.)[7]

Also related to his difficulties with eye-hand coordination, Hans takes a long time to dress himself, groom himself (including washing his hands) and eat. Whereas we know that this also is why he is sometimes late for school, Mrs. H. suggests that this also may be why Hans arrives late from lunch, and from the bathroom too. She also says that, unlike the other students, Hans needs help in hanging up his jacket and putting away his scarf and hat. She also observes that Hans covers his ears a lot, and thinks that it might have something to do with other children brushing against the carpeted floor, (but isn't sure).

The lunch time supervisor mentioned to us last Wednesday, (3/15) that Hans often spills foods and beverages on his clothes and onto the floor, and that he needs help to clean himself up. She also says that he is one of the last ones to leave the cafeteria, and that he sometimes forgets to take all of his things with him.

Additional concerns surround Hans's participation in recess and group sports. Mr. G. (the fifth grade teacher, who also serves as a playground supervisor) spoke with us last week (3/17), because of a dispute that apparently happened on the playground. This incident resulted in Hans being excluded from playing *wall ball* by the other boys, because they claimed that he was not "following the rules." Mr. G. acknowledged that Hans has always been a considerate boy with others, and wondered if this illness (or something else) might be affecting his participation in play and in other group activities.

Moreover, when we attended the class field trip to *Seal Beach* last week (3/10) as chaperones, we noticed that Hans was not keeping up with the other students, and that he required constant assistance from one of the adults in order to avoid tripping on the trail, and falling behind. Mrs. H. also shared her concerns with us about Hans's lack of "sure-footedness" during PE and recess activities, and said that Hans's poor ability to follow along during group games and sports results in his often "sitting out" on the class activity.

Of course, we are also concerned about the amount of time that Hans is missing from school. This is not only due to symptoms of the illness itself (such as fear of being separated from his mother, fatigue and headaches in the morning, and taking a long time to complete grooming activities), but also traveling to necessary doctor appointments. All of these significantly limit his participation and function in school.

Last, but not least, we are worried about the increase in Hans's facial tics (also associated with this illness), and are eager to know how we can address this, so that his participation in school activities do not suffer. Of course, we remain vigilant that such illness-related symptoms (that our son has no control over) do not result in his being a target of bullying or harassment, and so are eager to work with the school staff to address such eventualities if they occur. As everyone who has worked with him knows, Hans has always been a kind and caring boy who has easily gotten along with others. We do not want symptoms of this illness to begin to interfere with his social development and interaction with other students.

Based on these concerns, we request that, in keeping with federal laws regarding the assessment of all areas of suspected areas of disability, the school district conduct the following evaluations:[8]

1. A school nursing plan, so that the district nurse can evaluate and monitor aspects of Hans's nursing needs related to PANS and his education. Attached is the contact information from his treating provider, Dr. S., along with her letter that confirms his diagnosis and provides recommendations for the school.
2. A psycho-educational evaluation to determine Hans's present level of processing strengths and weaknesses, and to determine present levels of verbal and nonverbal intelligence.
3. Assessments to determine present levels of academic skills and achievement, such as in reading, math, and writing.
4. Evaluations by a registered Occupational Therapist to evaluate fine motor weaknesses, (including handwriting difficulties), levels of skills of daily living (including grooming, dressing, and eating), and to rule out, or confirm, sensory dysfunction and overwhelm (related to his poor balance and coordination on walks etc., and difficulty with handling certain sounds, respectively).

5. Evaluations by an Adapted Physical Education instructor to determine Hans's gross motor abilities (on his own, and also in a group activity). Moreover, Hans has said that he feels "like he has to move around a lot" in between Science and afternoon recess (*at which time he is in class for about an hour and a half, without a break*). Could the adapted physical education teacher (or the occupational therapist) advise Mrs. H. on brief activities he could do to stay awake and/or keep focused?
6. Evaluations by a Speech and Language Pathologist to determine (verbal *and* non-verbal) receptive and expressive language abilities, including oral motor abilities and articulation, etc.
7. Evaluations in the area of visual processing to determine Hans's abilities in the areas of visual analysis, discrimination, analysis/ synthesis, short term, long term, and working memory, visual-spatial orientation, and scanning.

Of special note, we have become aware that deficits in *visual processing skills* are often included among PANS symptoms. As we know that Hans has problems with eye-hand coordination, visual memory, and writing down what he is told (dictation), we want to make sure that he is given tests that measure his visual processing skills *separately* from his auditory and fine motor abilities, as well as *in combination* with them. We also believe that it is important to find out what his visual processing and fine motor skills are under *timed* and *untimed* conditions. As it is recognized by leading researchers who study PANS, that visual processing deficits are known to interfere in achievement and learning among affected students, we consider the assessment of Hans's visual processing abilities to be a critical piece in his evaluation. For this reason, we request that the following instruments be considered for use as part of his assessment:
The Wide Range Assessment of Memory and Learning (WRAML);
The Rey-Osterrieth Complex Figure Test (ROCF);
The 'Draw a Person' Test;
The Children's Memory Scale (Visual Memory Composite);
The 'Finger Tapping' Test; and
The Stroop Color-Word Interference Test.

We request that Hans be evaluated with the above tests (or their equivalent), as *these specific measures* were used in studies that examined neurocognitive functioning (deficiencies) in students with PANS.[9]
If a qualified examiner in visual processing deficits is not available within the school district, we request that the district provide Hans with an evaluation from the Binocular Vision Clinic at UC Stockton (which is a well-regarded teaching hospital in this field).[10]

8. Lastly, we request assessments to determine levels of Hans's social and emotional development, as it relates to any behaviors that may be seen at school and at home, and to gauge his current need, and type, of therapeutic counseling. We believe that recommendations drawn from these evaluations are needed to help Hans manage his symptoms and feelings at school (so that he can fully participate in the learning setting as much as possible).

Due to Hans's limited energy levels and attention span, we ask that he be evaluated for no longer than forty five minutes in any given testing session (where sitting down, listening, reading, writing, or other activities that require concentration are needed). Breaks will help to ensure that the testing results will be more valid, especially considering the taxing nature of his illness.

Moreover, in addition to the presence of the district registered nurse, Mrs. L. and the evaluating professionals listed above, we request that Mrs. H. (his teacher) attend this planning meeting, along with the 504 representative.

Lastly, as Mr. D. and I are needed to work at our farm in the morning, we request that any meeting begin after 1 pm. Due to the serious nature of our son's condition, we request that all timelines regarding assessments and meetings be met, not only within the procedural timelines provided by law, but preferably, before then.

If you have any questions or need to discuss this further, please call us at (349) 666-1124 or alternatively on my husband Oliver's cell phone (443) 484-2968.

Thanks in advance for your assistance.

Sincerely,

Lisa and Oliver D.

Notes

[1] Of course, it will be important to speak with the medical provider as well to discuss these academic issues and concerns.

[2] Home/Hospital instruction is a good example of how one needs to be aware of varying laws and educational codes that prevail where one lives. In some states, for example, a doctor's note will suffice to receive home instruction. In other states home/hospital instruction is covered under special education. and/or Section 504.

[3] Generally based on US education law.

[4] Or, alternatively, he is receiving testing or treatment to *rule/out PANS.*

[5] This is a very long letter, but will hopefully give the reader an idea of the types of things to include when requesting such services.

[6] Or, alternatively, he is receiving testing or treatment to *rule/out PANS.*

[7] Examples of known changes regard the student's ability to function or fully participate (in the classroom, in collaborative work groups with peers, on the playground, in PE, on field trips, etc.).

[8] *"(4) The child is assessed in all areas related to the suspected disability, including, if appropriate, health, vision, hearing, social and emotional status, general intelligence, academic performance, communicative status, and motor abilities"* from Regulations: Part 300 / D / 300.304; Sec. 300.304 *Evaluation procedures.* http://idea.ed.gov/explore/view/p/,root,regs,300,D,300%252E304, May,2015;

[9] One can *request* specific tests, but schools are not required to use those specific tests. They may use other tests that measure the same aspects of the disability, and that would be considered acceptable.

[10] Keep in mind that, whether or not the family or the school initiates services from a binocular vision clinic, etc. there are provisions (US) for the school district to pay for vision therapy, if it is directly related to the student's educational needs.

Appendix V: Goals and Objectives

The following examples are written to illustrate the parameters of appropriate goals and objectives in Special Education and in most educational plans.

Goals

When participants at educational meetings are considering *goals* for the student, they typically are thinking of what *growth* the student can be expected to make in a specific block of time. These goals surround academics, of course, but also *all areas of function and development* related to his or her disability. Often these goals are yearly goals, but in the case of a student with PANS, for example, goals can, and often should, be written for shorter periods of time. Note in the examples below, the goals are measurable, and based on what the student can actually demonstrate. Included also in the goal writing, is a summation of present level of performance, or baseline information.

Objectives

Objectives are measurable benchmarks towards the goal.

Examples of Goals and Objectives

Area of Need: Social Skills; *Baseline:* Seventh grader Hans D. falls behind with his academic work due to prolonged absences from school.

Measured Annual Goal: "By 9/24/16, Hans will increase his ability to function appropriately within the school environment, as measured by the benchmark or objective listed below."[1]

Example of an Objective: "By March 1 of 2015, Hans will independently indicate the need to take a break to go to the bathroom, by signaling with a visual placard to instructor 100% of the time, as measured by teacher records and weekly student feedback to case manager."

Strategies that will focus on Goals/ Objectives: Educational Team participants should understand how these goals and objectives will be taught. In the instance above, for example: a) One can assign a permanent bathroom pass to the student during the period of his illness. b) The instructor(s) will be notified that this will be used in their classes as well as advised (along with the student) on how to complete this transaction with as little disruption as possible.
c) The case manager or special education teacher should explain the parameters of the use of the bathroom pass, and where it is expected that the student should go (which bathroom or possibly rest area).
Another simple example would be where the goal involved physical development and sports activity.

Area of Need: Physical Development and Gross Motor Skills; Baseline: Seventh grader Hans D. currently has less than 10 percent participation in grade level minutes of physical education and sports activity, as indicated by attendance sheets.

Measured Annual Goal: "By 9/24/16, Hans will increase his walking skills by walking four times a week for fifteen minutes, as measured by record forms provided by the Adapted Physical Education teacher, and filled out by Hans and signed by Mrs. D."

Examples of objectives that would support or work towards this goal might include: "By 6/24/16, Hans will be able to verbally identify 3 indications of fatigue," or, "By 6/24/15, Hans will demonstrate the ability to do warm-up or cool-down techniques related to walking," or "By 6/03/15, Hans will demonstrate the ability to use proper breathing techniques related to walking, as measured by...."

Examples of IEP Goals without Objectives

In some instances, goals may be written without objectives. However, they still need to be measurable and specific. An example of such a goal would be the following:
With a goal in the area of third grade writing skills, a specific goal might be, "By April 1, 2016, and given direct instruction by the teacher, visual supports (task list), and using the class voice-to-text software "*Dragon Dictate*," Hans will demonstrate the ability to dictate, edit, and publish a four sentence paragraph, with less than two spelling errors per submitted text (4 out of 5 submissions)."

Statement of Needed Special Education and Other Services and Supports

Along with goals and objectives, there is also a provision under IDEA for a statement of needed special education and other services. These will include those supplementary aids, services (such as speech therapy) and other supports for school personnel to help this student, or for this student to use directly. This list would also include such information as *a start date, end date, frequency, duration, and location*. A few examples of these would be the following:

"<u>Service:</u> *Specialized Academic Instruction;* Provider: *Hinkley School, Ms. Martin;* Location of Service: *Room 491 (Ms. Martin's classroom)* Duration/Frequency: *282 minutes a week;* Start Date and End Date: *9/24/15-9/24/16."*

"<u>Service:</u> *Speech Therapy;* Provider: *Hinkley School, Ms. M.;* Location of Service: *Room 301;* Duration/Frequency: *45 minutes twice weekly.* Start Date and End Date: *9/24/15-9/24/16.*
Depending upon the forms that the district uses, other supports with checklists to include related identifiers regarding dates, minutes provided, and location, etc. may include:

> *"Provide lecture notes as needed."*
> *"Provide Hans with an alternate assignment for puzzles or crosswords."*
> *"Allow Hans extra time on tests and assignments as needed (up to 2X extra time)."*
> *"Teachers are asked to prioritize all work for Hans, allowing him to complete essential work only, not to exceed 2/3 of the work assigned."*
> *"Teachers are to refrain from asking Hans if he is listening in class."*
> *"Teachers are to redirect Han's focus by speaking to him after class, in private, and one-on-one."*

Regardless of the governmental or district oversight related to a particular school (or different forms that schools may use), a good educational plan is written so that interventions reflect the following: the student's disabling condition warrants such measures; there is accord among the team that such actions are appropriate; interventions are measurable in terms of effectiveness; and they are written to include *who* is doing the service, *where* and *when* is the intervention taking place, and for how long.

Notes

---

[1] Although only one example of an objective is listed for this goal, there can be a number of objectives listed for each goal.

CPSIA information can be obtained
at www.ICGtesting.com
Printed in the USA
LVOW05s2036040617
536902LV00014B/34/P